The Serotonin Solution

Also by Judith J. Wurtman:

EATING YOUR WAY THROUGH LIFE

THE CARBOHYDRATE CRAVER'S DIET

Coauthored by Judith J. Wurtman:

THE CARBOHYDRATE CRAVER'S COOKBOOK

MANAGING YOUR MIND AND MOOD THROUGH FOOD

The Serotonin Solution

**JUDITH J. WURTMAN, Ph.D.
and SUSAN SUFFES**

Fawcett Columbine
New York

To my granddaughters Dvora and Yael

The Massachusetts Institute of Technology owns patents on use of dexfenfluramine for treating obesity, carbohydrate craving, smoking withdrawal, PMS, and SAD. These patents have been licensed to the Servier Co. in Neuilly-sur-Seine, France. The patent for obesity has been sublicensed to an American company, Interneron, Inc. The author, Judith J. Wurtman, is the co-inventor of these patents and is an advisor to Interneron, Inc., and owns stock in this company.

However, the views on dietary and pharmacological therapy expressed in this book are solely those of the author. No company has approved, endorsed, or sponsored this book, and any brand-name references are factual and are included for informational purposes only.

The subject matter described in certain portions of this book, in particular, Chapter Five ("The Serotonin-Seeker's Diet"), is covered by a pending application for patent with the United States Patent and Trademark Office. The sale of this book does not include an express or implied license to practice the invention disclosed in the pending application for patent.

Thou shalt eat and be satisfied.

—DEUTERONOMY 11:15

CONTENTS

FOREWORD

For over fifteen years my colleagues and I at the Massachusetts Institute of Technology have been conducting research on how our eating is affected by our emotional state. During that time I have also worked with hundreds of overweight men and women who come to MIT to participate in our clinical weight-loss programs. Many are at the end of their ropes after years of dieting failures. They feel that they'll never be able to stop the overeating that spells doom to even their most determined attempts at weight control. After many studies, the pieces to the puzzle have fallen into place. We now have a clear picture of the relationship of emotional state and appetite. It is apparent that stress-induced overeating is not a problem of lack of willpower or restraint but is caused by changes in the brain system that regulates our mood and our appetite. I call this system the stress-management system. The key to it is the brain chemical "serotonin." Serotonin's activity keeps our emotions and eating under control. When serotonin is not able to function normally due to stress, the result is often an uncontrolled emotional state and bingeing.

Several years ago, I discovered through studies carried out at MIT's Clinical Research Center that serotonin's activity could be restored by eating the right foods—specifically, carbohydrate foods that don't contain much fat. High-carbohydrate diets composed of carefully regulated amounts of protein and carbohydrates eaten according to a fixed schedule had a biochemical impact on the brain and made volunteers feel a sense of emotional well-being, which in turn significantly reduced the food cravings that routinely caused them to overeat whether or not they were physically hungry. A similar improvement occurred when volunteers were treated with dexfenfluramine, a drug that increases the activity of serotonin.

Until recently, the exciting results of our research have been known only to those who read about it in scientific journals and to patients who come to me for counseling. *The Serotonin Solution* makes this information available to you. This book will help you if you are one of the millions of people who overeat when stressed. *The Serotonin Solution* contains food plans I've developed at MIT designed to help you stop bingeing and lose weight. And, you'll experience a greater sense of calm and well-being than you've experienced on any other reducing diet you've ever tried. The food plans can be used by

- those of you who want to lose weight but cannot do so successfully because your diet collapses as soon as you experience emotional distress
- those of you who worry about gaining back the weight you have lost on diets, because when you try to eat normally, emotions destroy your control over your eating
- those of you who are holding on to your control over eating by a thread even though your weight is not a problem

The food plans can also be used by themselves or along with serotonin-activating prescription weight-loss medications, including dexfenfluramine, more commonly known under the brand name Redux. The food plans will enhance the efficiency of these drugs if followed during treatment and will allow you to continue to lose weight or maintain the weight you have lost after you stop taking the drug.

As effective as the food plans are, *The Serotonin Solution* is not for everyone. The food plans do reduce emotional stress, but they are not a substitute for therapies for clinical disorders such as depression, bulimia, anxiety disorders, and obsessive-compulsive disorder. They should not be used by anyone with a metabolic disorder that requires a special dietary regimen, such as diabetes. The information, suggestions, and guidelines presented in this book are not intended to replace professional medical advice. You should consult with your physician prior to and during participation in this or any other weight-loss program. And the food plans will probably not be relevant for those few of you who tend to lose weight when you are upset.

But for those of you who have up until now felt that your attempts to lose weight and keep it off were fruitless because stress always made you fail, *The Serotonin Solution* is the solution to your overeating problems.

ACKNOWLEDGMENTS

This book would not have been written without the support and efforts of many people. The first is my husband, Richard, whose scientific insights and creativity fueled much of the research that generated this book. Although our discussions about science were more likely to occur at the dinner table than the conference table (and once on the top of a mountain in Switzerland), they resulted in many years of exciting and successful studies on the relationship between the brain, emotions, and overeating. Without his support as a partner in all my endeavors, I would not have been able to write the book.

I must also mention those individuals whose research contributions and friendship made this book possible. I am especially grateful to Janine McDermott, the research coordinator on all of our MIT studies. Her unfailing good humor and patience and ability always to find the crucial piece of paper and rescue me from my inevitable fights with the computer has made our many years of working together a joy and delight. I am also indebted to Rita Tsay, whose role as research dietitian has been crucial in the design and implementation of our projects. Life in our research unit would be very dull without our daily discussions (arguments?) over some aspect of an ongoing study or simply the chance to talk.

My trainer and friend, Bill Corcoran, was the source of much of the information on exercise. Although much of it was imparted while I was struggling with yet another bicep curl or chest press, his mini-lectures on the most effective types of exercise and warnings about exercise fads and equipment that are either useless or potentially harmful were invaluable. And I will never forget his admonition to make the writing of this book my first priority while I was struggling to handle many competing demands.

I will always be indebted to Susan Suffes, my co-author, whose laughter and funny stories brightened the weeks and weeks of rewriting and on whom I knew I could always rely to pull us through a difficult revision. Virginia Faber, my editor, comes in for special thanks as well. Despite a frantically tight schedule, she allowed me to make changes I felt were necessary up to the last minute and smoothed the entire writing and publication process. Moreover, she even went beyond the call of editorial duty by testing successfully the calming effect of carbohydrate in the middle of last-minute Christmas shopping.

And finally, I want to acknowledge my literary agent, Linda Chester, who supported the idea of the book from its initial tentative beginnings. She made the book happen. Thank you, Linda, for your belief in the concept and your unfailing cheerfulness and resourcefulness whenever any problem arose.

CHAPTER ONE

Stress: The Villain Behind the Numbers on the Scale

For many of us, the impulse to reach for something to eat when we are upset seems as natural and inevitable as breathing. Who among us has never gobbled up a candy bar, a handful of cookies, or a fistful of nuts when we are feeling stressed? The angry phone call from a relative we've unwittingly offended, the confrontation with a spouse or teenagers, the leak in the roof when our finances are strained, the dent in your new car, the lost house keys, an unexpected bill—these situations are but some of the kinds of daily attacks that can undermine our attempts to control our eating.

Does this sound familiar? You've had a really rough day. The kids fought from the moment they woke up until they went to school, you were late getting to work, the deal you were working on fell through, and your nerves are jangling like a wind chime in a hurricane. Your reaction involves consuming a giant-size bag of almond M&M's.

Or perhaps you are dreading the coming holidays because any prolonged contact with your family dredges up decades of unresolved conflicts. So you deal with your anxiety by eating yourself sick, giving the Thanksgiving turkey stiff competition in the stuffing department.

Or maybe you recognize this scenario. The man you've been dating for three months suddenly starts doing a disappearing act—forgetting the theater date you had been looking forward to, canceling the weekend you had planned together, asking for a rain check on dinner. Maybe he really is overworked, as he claims, or maybe he's bailing out. You know you should keep busy seeing other people, doing all the things you usually enjoy, but the only activity that appeals to you now involves lifting a fork weighted down with pasta in cream sauce to your mouth while sitting in front of the television. You can't stop eating—not until he calls again.

WHY WE OVEREAT

For most people, overeating triggered by some variety of emotional distress is the demon behind the ever-escalating numbers we see on the scale. Every day we promise to "be good," to eat only healthful foods, to count fat grams, and to exercise for at least thirty minutes three times a week. Yet every day we find ourselves gulping handfuls of candy, munching bag after bag of potato chips, or eating a quart of ice cream. We engage in this behavior for any number of reasons: anger, anxiety, depression, worry, frustration, loneliness, or emotional exhaustion.

And so our eating goes out of control and we feel helpless. As we contemplate the hundreds—sometimes even thousands—of calories we've ingested out of emotional need, we ask ourselves, "What is wrong with me? Haven't I one shred of willpower? Am I forever destined to be overweight?"

This is what Sally thought about herself when she told me her story, one of hundreds of similar stories I have heard in the last ten years. "This is what I looked like sixty pounds ago," Sally told me, showing me an oft-handled photo of herself as a sleek size eight in a bathing suit, quite a different person from the very unhappy size sixteen woman in front of me.

"It took me more than one year of rigorous dieting and exercising to get to my target weight—and less than six months to gain it back. And I certainly knew the drill: weigh and measure the food, read labels, cut out fat, throw out leftovers, call a friend for support or take a walk when you feel a binge coming on, get lots of exercise. I could have taught the behavioral-modification classes.

"But they don't teach you how to eat when your mother has a stroke, and you are the one responsible for getting her into a nursing home, dealing with the paperwork, selling her apartment, and feeling guilty that you can't move her in with you.

"So I ate. My best friend was the refrigerator. Every day I promised myself a well-balanced, nutritious meal, and every night I ate junk instead. I know if I had just had some willpower and self-discipline I would have been able to control my eating. Now my situation feels totally hopeless, and I don't think I'll ever be able to do anything about it."

Weight gain driven by emotional distress has turned Sally and millions of others like her into health statistics. According to a National Institutes of Health (NIH) report issued in 1992, a staggering 99 percent of all dieters put all their lost weight back on within five years of completing a diet program. The reason given by the NIH experts was accurate as far as it went but not very helpful in terms of our understanding what goes wrong—lack of compliance with the dietary and exercise guidelines for weight maintenance. Sally was well aware she was not following medically sound suggestions to monitor her portion size; eat low-fat foods; increase her consumption of fruits, vegetables, grain, and high-fiber products; and exercise. What she did not know was *why* she could not adhere to all the recommendations that had made her weight-loss attempts such an initial success. So she blamed herself, believing it was a fatal lack of self-discipline that was dooming her to life as a fat person.

When I asked her how she was able to stay on the diet program long enough to lose the sixty pounds, she told me that it really hadn't been all that hard. During those fourteen months, her life was relatively under control. Her mother had been healthy, and Sally had been working at a job she enjoyed that still gave her plenty of time to plan her meals and to exercise, and she'd had plenty of social opportunities to take pleasure in her ever-more-slender figure.

"Now," she related, "between my mother and my job I am wrung dry by the demands made upon me. I'm painfully aware that I'm eating as a reaction to the stress I am under. But I don't seem able to stop."

EMOTIONAL CONTROL = EATING CONTROL

When our emotions overwhelm us, we often turn to food to try to assuage them. Stress generates a powerful psychological hunger that never seems satisfied, no matter how full our stomachs feel. Stress is the culprit that makes us ignore food that is good for us and yearn for the cookies, candy, or ice cream we know is bad. Stress causes us to throw away the hard-earned results of weeks or months of careful eating and disciplined exercise regimens. Stress makes us drive through a middle-of-the-night rainstorm to a twenty-four-hour convenience store for a box of glazed dough-nuts or pull a frozen cake from the freezer and eat it before it thaws.

It's not so hard to understand why the behavior-modification lessons we learned in many diet programs don't work to prevent our overeating under stress. Who among us can remember to eat slowly, chew our food thoroughly, or put our forks down between bites, when the only thing that's holding back our howls of frustration and misery is a full mouth? How many of us have the discipline or self-control to get on a treadmill or ride a bike when we feel overwhelmed by sadness or worry? All the best advice in the world on how to control our food intake and engage in regular physical activity becomes irrelevant when we are the victims of stress. At those times—and they come with great regularity—the only relief we feel is when we eat.

A friend of mine tried desperately to maintain a sensible

eating and exercise routine for several months while enduring an extremely frustrating situation in her career. Laid off
from an excellent managerial job when her company down-
sized, she resolved to follow the diet and exercise regimen that
had helped her to lose pounds successfully earlier that year. After all, looking good was more important than ever, now that
she was back on the job market. As time passed and job offers
did not materialize, she found herself less and less able to control her eating. Eventually she simply gave up and sat home,
eating her way through several more months of unemploy-
ment. Numerous jars of peanut butter spread on countless
loaves of bread caused her to gain almost thirty pounds. But as
much as she would have liked to stop, she couldn't: Eating was
the only activity that seemed to soothe her ever-increasing anxiety over her joblessness.

Emotionally driven eating is an unavoidable response to real
life. When we are feeling stressed, our urge to overeat doesn't go
away. It can't. This is because the force that drives us to put food
in our mouths when we are stressed is biological. Denying it only
causes it to grow stronger, delay further intensifies it, and stifling
it ultimately propels it to break loose. The result can be an eating
free-for-all—in other words, a binge.

Are You an Impulsive Overeater?

Often, overeating patterns are so ingrained we don't realize we
have them, and our personal "triggers," that is, the particular
emotional stresses that cause us to lose control of our eating, are
so common that we don't recognize them as such. Ask yourself,
"Do I overeat . . ."

1. when I feel fatigued?
2. during business meals because I am worried about making a
good impression?
3. when I have difficulty falling asleep?
4. after my weekly meeting with my boss?

5. right before I get my period?
6. to keep myself awake?
7. to put myself back to sleep in the middle of the night?
8. out of boredom?
9. when I am angry and do not want to show it?
10. when I feel like smoking a cigarette?
11. after an argument?
12. when I study for a big exam?
13. when I am writing something and have problems thinking of what to say?
14. as a way of procrastinating?
15. in social situations when I feel uncomfortable?
16. when I have lost something important and can't find it?
17. when I am alone and feeling lonely?
18. when I am left alone in the kitchen to clean up after dinner and everyone else is relaxing?
19. right before I go on a diet?
20. right after I go off a diet?
21. as a way of distracting myself from disturbing thoughts?
22. when I hate the way I look?
23. after I have gained back some of the weight I lost on a diet?
24. when I have to buy a dress for a wedding and everything looks awful?
25. instead of getting into an argument?
26. when I am nervous about being with people?
27. when I have too many things to do at the same time and have no help?
28. when I can't control a situation I know is spinning out of control?
29. when it is dark and gloomy outside?
30. on Sundays?
31. after a bad date?
32. when I see my relatives or those of my spouse?
33. after I have deprived myself of something I wanted to eat?

There probably isn't anybody who won't answer yes to at least some of the questions on this list. It is a rare person indeed who is not susceptible to impulsive, or emotion-driven, overeating. So if you found yourself saying yes over and over again as you read through the list, at least you will realize you are not alone. You and countless others like you are vulnerable to the effects of stress, and one major indicator of stress is overeating.

Your problem is not lack of willpower or self-discipline. Rather, you are the victim of your biological makeup. The overeating you cannot seem to control is caused by changes that take place in your brain when you are upset. Neither willpower nor self-discipline will work forever to stop the eating that occurs in response to these brain changes.

The good news is that there is a solution to the emotionally propelled overeating that adds unwanted pounds. And the answer has nothing to do with willpower, diets, behavioral modification, or gene therapy. Ironically, it is *food* that can best bring emotion-driven overeating under control.

CARBOHYDRATES

Food has a powerful effect on serotonin, a chemical in the brain that controls both emotion and eating. But it's not just any food that has this effect; it's food in the form of sweet or starchy carbohydrates.

Carbohydrates come in two basic varieties: sugars, which are also classified as simple carbohydrates; and starches, which are classified as complex carbohydrates. "Simple" and "complex" refer to the number and arrangement of the molecules that make up the structure of the carbohydrates. Sugars have a simpler molecular structure than starches.

Simple Carbohydrates: Sugars

The simplest carbohydrate is glucose, or dextrose, which is usually found in food in combination with another much sweeter sugar, fructose. Fructose and glucose combined form sucrose, or table sugar. Fructose, also known as fruit sugar, occurs naturally alone or in combination with glucose in fruits, honey, and maple syrup. Lactose is the sugar found in milk. It is composed of two smaller sugar molecules: glucose and galactose.

All these simple carbohydrates are sweet tasting, and, except for glucose, are used to flavor many of our foods. Honey, corn sweeteners that contain a combination of fructose and glucose, pancake and waffle syrups, and table sugar are common sweetening agents in commercial products and at home.

Complex Carbohydrates: Starches

Glucose molecules combined into long, branching chains are known as starches, or complex carbohydrates. Some of the starchy foods that are familiar to us include flour, grains, rice, corn, potatoes, winter squashes, barley, buckwheat groats, and oatmeal, as well as more exotic grains such as quinoa and amaranth.

Both sugars and starches are fat free in their natural states. However, they are very often cooked, processed, or combined with fat. It is the low-fat or fat-free version of carbohydrates, and specifically of the complex carbohydrates, that will be of particular use to you in the numerous diet plans I have included in this book. (The problems with fat will be explained in Chapter Two.)

PHYSICAL VERSUS PSYCHOLOGICAL HUNGER

For the past fifteen years my colleagues and I have been carrying out studies at the Clinical Research Center at the Massachusetts Institute of Technology. This research center, which is supported by the National Institutes of Health, carries out numerous studies on human volunteers, men and women who either live at the center while a study is conducted or come to the research facility as outpatients. Our staff members include physicians, nurses, dietitians, and psychologists, as well as other kinds of experts and specialists when warranted. I myself am a biochemist and the head of the Nutrition and Behavior Studies Group at the Clinical Research Center and a research scientist in the department of Brain and Cognitive Science at MIT. The center's research projects range from studies on memory, metabolism, mineral requirements, sleep therapies, and brain imaging (in collaboration with other research institutions in the area) to the effects of diet and drugs on food intake, weight changes, and behavior. My colleagues and I have carried out a number of studies over the past fifteen years on how serotonin affects our emotional state and our eating patterns, and how our emotional state and what we eat affects serotonin.

The conclusion of my research, based on studies of volunteers with many types of stress-driven overeating, is that there are two types of hunger: physical hunger, which is driven by our body's need for nourishment, and psychological hunger, which is propelled by our need for comfort and solace.

Physical hunger can be satisfied by eating a large variety of foods that supply not only calories but also necessary nutrients. But psychological hunger can only be relieved by eating foods that renew and restore serotonin. These foods consist specifically of sweet or starchy carbohydrates, either alone or in combination, that can include everything from candy, doughnuts, cake, cookies, cupcakes, frosting, and muffins to popcorn, bagels, potatoes, cornflakes, rice, tortillas, and pasta.

Once these foods enter the body and are digested, not only do they nourish us but they also have dramatic effects on our brains. Carbohydrates set off a series of biochemical events that result in the brain making serotonin and then activating the brain chemical to run our brain's stress-management system. This system soothes our emotional turmoil and, by doing so, stops the urge to binge. Eating carbohydrates is the only way to boost serotonin levels in the brain—because even if serotonin could be put in a pill and swallowed, it cannot get into the brain from the bloodstream. For this reason carbohydrates are considered a "psychoactive" food. When they are eaten in the correct "dose" and without other foods that might interfere with their effect, they have the power to bring about substantial changes in our mood.

Psychological hunger can be generated by any number of different kinds of stress. Most commonly it's the stresses of daily life that cause us to feel the need to eat when we're not hungry. Research at MIT has found that many of us routinely suffer from day-in day-out upheavals that result in regular cravings for certain kinds of food. But other situations also result in this kind of hunger, including premenstrual syndrome, which causes monthly changes in mood and appetite; the long dark days of winter, which for some people result in a syndrome called Seasonal Affective Disorder (SAD); smoking withdrawal; work schedules that run counter to normal sleeping/waking cycles; the minute-to-minute demands of caring for young children full-time; and even dieting itself or its aftermath.

All these situations are stressful and result in what I call psychological hunger. And it is this specific hunger—a carbohydrate-craving, serotonin-seeking drive—that must be satisfied in order to control emotional-based overeating.

But why does the brain translate the intricate biochemical signals associated with inadequate amounts of serotonin into a desire to eat jelly doughnuts? The easiest way to explain how this happens is to compare our cravings for carbohydrates with our need to drink when we are thirsty. Think about a hot day when you are gardening, doing chores, or taking a long walk. Inevitably you get very thirsty. Instinctively you know that you need to drink something that will work fast, and that sweet beverages like fruit juice or salty ones like soup won't do the job as effectively as water. Moreover, the longer you wait before drinking the more intense your thirst becomes. It will not go away, because it can't. If you are unable to satisfy your thirst immediately and keep on getting more and more dehydrated, you may eventually find yourself gulping glass after glass of water, actually "bingeing" on the liquid. But then, suddenly, the thirst is gone. Without any need to tell yourself to do so, you simply stop drinking. You did not have to think about stopping, use willpower, or employ any behavior-modification techniques. Your body, provided with enough water, simply told you to stop giving it any more.

What happened here? You felt thirsty because the brain sent signals, via hormones, that blood volume was down and you needed to drink liquids to bring it back to an acceptable level. Once the thirst was satisfied a feeling of great comfort replaced the intense drive that urged you to drink. You certainly never felt any concern about whether you would be able to stop drinking once you started. Nor would you ever consider yourself weak-willed or out of control because you responded to your thirst by drinking.

A similar series of events occurs when the brain is "thirsty" for serotonin. Suddenly you feel a nagging need to put something in your mouth, a need that will not go away. Willpower is helpless against it. You may try the distraction techniques learned in a behavior-modification class, but the biologically based hunger remains. That need for serotonin presents itself in a very specific way: It calls for a sweet or starchy food. You might try to satisfy it with an apple or a container of yogurt, but that serotonin thirst continues to demand what it wants. Inevitably you give in to the relentless nagging and grab a sweet or starchy snack. And by doing so you satisfy your serotonin "thirst." Just as you automatically stop drinking water when your body has enough, if you eat the correct amount of carbohydrates and wait the appropriate amount of time, the need to eat simply evaporates. Your desperate need for serotonin has been satisfied.

But why, if we do not drink more than we need when we are thirsty, do we often eat more than necessary when we are desperately seeking serotonin?

The answer has to do with the relative speed with which thirst, as opposed to hunger, can be satisfied. Because water or other liquids race through our intestinal tract and into our bloodstream within a few minutes of our drinking them, our brain almost immediately receives a signal that water is entering the body. When enough water enters, a complex set of hormones is activated that decreases our perception of thirst.

However, the passage of food through our digestive tract takes much longer. The passage from the mouth to the part of the small intestine where foods that are digested can enter the bloodstream is a long, slow trip, and the biochemical processes that need to occur before serotonin production can begin take yet more time.

When we are desperately seeking serotonin, we eat more and more food, often very quickly, until our stomach fills up and stretches to the point of feeling pain. Unfortunately, for reasons I will explain in subsequent chapters, we can eat prodigious amounts of potato chips, ice cream, or pasta before the biochemical events that lead to serotonin production in the brain occur.

The Serotonin Solution will explain how to eat to speed the production of serotonin and satisfy your particular kind of psychological hunger, whether it's caused by the stresses of daily life, PMS, SAD, smoking withdrawal, night-shift work, full-time mothering, or dieting. The food plans in this book—one for each of the conditions named—are based on years of published research carried out at MIT in which my colleagues and I measured, biochemically and behaviorally, the effects of food on the brain. Because of our work I have come to the conclusion that sweet and starchy foods act as a natural medication. When consumed in the right dose according to the appropriate schedule, carbohydrates can prime our serotonin stress-management system, putting us back in control of our emotions and our eating.

THE FOOD PLANS

You won't have to engage in guesswork to figure out which food plan best suits your psychological hunger, because in Chapter Four I've provided questionnaires to enable you to identify your particular stress triggers. For many people it's just the ups and downs of daily life that keep the best of intentions from becoming reality. Or perhaps you are an overeater only during the winter months, easily reverting to normal eating during summer. Perhaps you never had a problem with bingeing until you decided to stay at home and become a full-time mother. Maybe you recently started to do shift work and find that you are eating both to stay awake *and* go to sleep. Or you could be like many people coming off a successful diet who find that they lose control of their eating once the program is over. For many women it's the monthly hormonal changes of PMS that throw their normally good eating habits into a tailspin. And then there are the smokers who have just kicked the habit and are now facing the cravings that so often lead to weight gain in those first cigaretteless months.

Each food plan in this book is unique, because different kinds of stress result in different kinds of overeating and different demands on your serotonin levels and activity. All the plans can be used to control impulsive overeating, whether or not you have a weight problem. But most of the plans are geared toward weight loss, on the assumption that if you have a problem with overeating you have a weight problem too. All the plans make sure you eat carbohydrate-rich foods in amounts sufficient to maintain serotonin levels and activity while you are losing weight. The plans differ from one another in three ways: when you eat the carbohydrates, what types of carbohydrates you should eat, and how much carbohydrate you need to consume. These variables are keyed to the biochemistry of the different stressors.

You can switch from one plan to another as your stress levels and emotional and eating needs change. If you suffer from PMS, then you will want to follow the PMS weight-loss plan in Chapter Seven for however long your symptoms last each month. If you move from southern California to northern Vermont, where the winter days are short, dark, and gloomy, you might find yourself experiencing a weight gain in December, January, and February. The seasonal plans in Chapter Eight will help you to minimize weight gain in the winter and maximize weight loss in the spring and summer. Of course, if you decide to move back to sunnier climates and still need to lose weight, you can switch back to the basic diet plan in Chapter Five.

Most of the plans will allow you to lose a slow but constant amount of weight, ranging from one to two pounds a week. This is a medically recommended rate of weight loss that protects you from losing muscle mass along with fat. Preserving muscle mass is very important, because it is your muscles that use up most of the calories you consume. The less muscle mass you have, the fewer calories you will be able to eat without regaining pounds after the diet is over.

Any of the plans can be followed even if you do not have to lose weight. Maintenance may be your goal. If you want to control emotion-driven overeating and decrease stress, then follow the basic outlines of the food plan you choose. Maintain the proportions of carbohydrates relative to protein, and adhere to the recommendations for lowering your fat intake, but increase the total amount of food you eat each day so that the calorie count goes up by 600 to 1,000 more per day for a total of 1,800 to 2,400 calories. (The number of calories you should eat will depend on your size, metabolism, and daily energy expenditure.)

All the plans in this book will work to boost your serotonin levels and activity, to satisfy your psychological hunger, and to bring both your eating and emotions under control. All the plans employ brainpower—not willpower—to help you lose weight and keep it off.

There is a separate chapter for each of the seven different problem areas we've identified in our research. You'll find:

- a daily stress-relief diet plan that keeps your levels of serotonin high throughout the day so you will always have ample stores of this potent brain chemical to draw upon when you really need it—which could be at any moment
- two premenstrual-syndrome food plans (one is chocolate-coated) that are customized to satisfy the specific mood and appetite changes that occur each month
- a seasonally adjusted food plan that prevents weight gain during the long dark days of winter and accelerates weight loss during the bright sunny days of summer
- an ex-smoker's food plan that compensates for nicotine damage to your eating-control system

- Mommy-stress food plans that calm and control eating even on the most intense days with preschool children
- a shift-worker's food plan tailored for the eating, sleeping, and weight loss needs of those who work while the rest of us are asleep
- an after-diet food plan specifically designed to restore serotonin and eating control destroyed by conventional diets

IT'S ALL IN YOUR MIND—
BUT NOT THE WAY YOU THINK

I know that many of you think that the only way to control your eating is to stay away entirely from the carbohydrates you continually crave. Experience has taught you that once you put something sweet or starchy in your mouth, it triggers a binge. You don't believe that you can rely on an internal control system to manage your overeating. Experience has taught you that the only way you can stick to a diet is to rely on external controls: Join a program, be weighed every week, and have someone monitor your food intake closely.

You *can* rely on yourself. You do have the brainpower to control your eating. The serotonin stress-management system has the potential to operate as effectively in your brain as in the skinniest person you know. This system will control your overeating even when you are bombarded by stress. But like a car whose oil or gas reserves are near empty, the serotonin stress-management system will not work if its serotonin stores are too low to meet the demands made upon it. Eating carbohydrates in the correct dose and at the correct time is the only way to ensure that your brain can take charge of your eating.

Doreen was typical of many so-called compulsive eaters who told us that once she started eating anything sweet, she couldn't stop. She was extremely skeptical of our program that required eating high-carbohydrate meals and snacks, certain she would binge. The opposite happened. When she came to see us after two weeks on the serotonin-seekers diet, she complained about having too much to eat. "I'm never hungry," she told us, as if hunger were a necessary by-product of dieting. "Why do I have to eat so much?" When we reminded her that lack of hunger hadn't stopped her overeating in the past, she said, "You're right. The diet has taken away my need to constantly pick at food when I am upset or worried."

In *The Serotonin Solution* I have converted the results of our research into food plans that will satisfy your psychological hunger, maintain the brain's reservoir of serotonin, and stimulate your stress-management system to manage your eating. Stress will no longer stimulate impulsive overeating. And you won't need superhuman willpower. The only "deprivation" you will experience is eating less fat. As you will read in Chapter Two, fat is not the answer to satisfying your psychological hunger, even though most of the comfort foods you seek are very high in fat. After you read about how fat affects your brain and emotional state, you will understand why you need to avoid high-fat foods when you want fast stress relief.

Many of you may either already be taking or may be considering treatment with serotonin-activating weight-loss medications, including the widely prescribed fen-fen combination and the newly approved drug dexfenfluramine, more commonly known by its brand name Redux. These drugs are successful in removing the desire to overeat by making you feel both physically and psychologically full. But they don't work in a vacuum. While they enhance serotonin activity in the brain, they have no effect on the brain's supply of serotonin. To maximize the drugs' effectiveness you should follow a diet that maintains optimal levels of serotonin. The food plans in this book will work to augment a drug treatment program, whether you are on the drug for a few months or several years, because they are designed to keep serotonin levels high. Once you have completed your therapy with the drug, the diet plans will allow you to continue to lose weight if this is still your goal, or help you maintain the weight loss you have achieved.

In the next chapter I will explain how and why the scientific principles that underlie the food plans can work to control stress-induced overeating. You will learn how serotonin acts in the brain to restore emotional well-being and to put the brake on excessive eating. And you will learn how to use food to boost your serotonin production so that eating will no longer veer out of control, regardless of the type of stress you are enduring.

CHAPTER TWO

Your Serotonin Stress-Management System: The Brain Behind the Binge

Anyone who has ever found herself ripping open a bag of chocolate chips and eating them by the handful or polishing off leftover pie at 3 A.M. by the light of the open refrigerator door is familiar with the following litany of questions. Why am I doing this to myself? Why am I devouring this chocolate cake when earlier in the day I carefully removed the inside of a bagel to cut down on calories? Why am I wolfing down this Danish when my stomach is still stuffed from the huge dinner I ate last night and I'm not even hungry?

The answer lies in our brains, specifically in the chemical serotonin. When we experience an uncontrollable urge to eat as a result of stress—and specifically to eat carbohydrates—it is because the serotonin in our brain is not functioning adequately.

Because the noninvasive techniques needed to assess brain changes are still being developed, scientists are not exactly sure what happens to serotonin during stress. Perhaps too little of it is made to meet increased demands, or stress causes it to be used up faster than usual, or the cells that react to serotonin become for some reason less responsive than usual and therefore demand larger quantities of this brain chemical. Fortunately, it is not necessary to know exactly what happens to serotonin in the brain to know how these changes affect you. All you need to know is one vital piece of information: Emotional distress affects serotonin, and for many of us this results in an overwhelming desire to eat.

THE SEROTONIN-STRESS AND CARBOHYDRATE-SEROTONIN CONNECTIONS

How is serotonin connected to our emotions and our appetites? About forty years ago scientists who worked on the association between the brain and psychological disturbances like depression noted that serotonin and a number of other brain chemicals, which are known as neurotransmitters because they transmit signals from one brain cell to another, were involved in regulating our moods.

Serotonin was one of the key neurotransmitters that seemed to malfunction in people who were stressed, anxious, depressed, tense, irritable, confused, angry, or mentally fatigued. When people suffering from these mood disturbances were treated with drugs that increased the activity of serotonin in the brain, they felt better. Their depression lessened, and they became calmer, less angry, more focused, energetic, and relaxed. Prozac, Zoloft, Paxil, and Effexor are some of the newest drugs developed to activate serotonin when it appears to be functioning abnormally because of a variety of emotional disturbances.

But what was the connection between feeling down in the dumps, annoyed, or irritated and craving potato chips, crackers, or chocolate? Did these commonplace mood changes also involve serotonin? And if so why do so many of us feel the need to eat when bad moods strike?

Finding the answer to these questions took over fifteen years of research at MIT and at other research facilities as well, in collaboration with a variety of colleagues. The individual with whom I have worked most and who was responsible for stimulating my interest in researching this question is my husband, Richard

Wurtman, a medical doctor, director of MIT's Clinical Research Center, and MIT's Cecil H. Green Distinguished Professor.

In the 1970s he and one of his graduate students, John Fernstrom, who is now a professor at the University of Pittsburgh, discovered the relationship between carbohydrate consumption and serotonin production. In a series of studies in which rats were fed a diet containing mostly starch and sugar and very small amounts of protein, they found that tryptophan, an amino acid (one of the building blocks of protein), was rapidly entering the brain. Earlier research had shown that serotonin was made from tryptophan and that as soon as levels of tryptophan in the brain increased, serotonin synthesis would also increase. As the cells accumulated new serotonin, it would be used immediately for the brain function that required its presence. When Wurtman and Fernstrom examined the brains of the rats after they ate a sweet or starchy meal, they found increased amounts of serotonin as well as increased activity in the systems that use serotonin.

None of this happened when the rats ate moderate amounts of protein along with the carbohydrates, a finding they did not understand at first. Eventually Wurtman and Fernstrom, along with others doing research in this area, learned that eating protein prevents tryptophan from entering the brain. It appeared that tryptophan has to compete with other similarly shaped amino acids for entry to the brain. All of these amino acids share a similar cellular passageway through the membrane that surrounds the brain. Tryptophan is at a disadvantage because it is found in smaller amounts in protein than all the other amino acids. After the protein-rich foods the rats ate were digested the blood became flooded with the amino acids that compete with tryptophan for "space" in the entryway into the brain. So when Wurtman and Fernstrom examined the brains of rats who had eaten protein along with the sweet and starchy carbohydrates, they found very little of this amino acid and very little newly made serotonin.

What remained to be learned was how eating carbohydrates, which do *not* contain tryptophan, can result in a brain full of this amino acid. The answer lies in the activity of insulin, a hormone secreted by the pancreas whenever we eat carbohydrates. Normally blood contains tryptophan and the other twenty-one amino acids in fairly constant amounts. After your body digests carbohydrates, insulin enters the bloodstream to push glucose, the digested form of carbohydrates, into the cells where it can be used for energy. During this process insulin also pushes amino acids circulating in the blood into the muscle cells. For reasons we don't yet completely understand, insulin leaves tryptophan behind in the bloodstream, where it is free to enter the brain. Both simple and complex carbohydrates will cause this rearrangement of amino acids in the bloodstream with the exception of fructose, the sugar found in fruits. Fructose has to be converted into glucose by the liver before insulin can be secreted and as a result so little insulin is released that it does not remove enough of the competing amino acids from the bloodstream.

My colleagues and I discovered that when individuals suffering from stress and mood disturbances ate carbohydrates, their dispositions improved and they no longer experienced the depressed, anxious, tense, irritable, confused, angry feelings and fatigue associated with stress. The second critical observation we made was that stress and its associated moods provoked a *hunger* for sweet or starchy carbohydrates. In other words, the body knows what the brain needs, and it demands it—sometimes with great urgency.

This is how we believe the brain's stress-management system works. (Confirmation awaits better techniques for studying how the chemicals in the brain interact to monitor emotional states.) Prolonged periods of stress, regardless of the cause, increase the brain's need for serotonin. How does the brain get more serotonin? We know that it can be made only when enough tryptophan is available. Therefore, the brain responds by sending out subtle signals that cause you to feel an impulse to eat something sweet or starchy. You respond by eating cookies, cake, cereal, or anything that contains a lot of sugar or starch or both.

The carbohydrate food is then digested, insulin is released, and the rapid depletion of all the amino acids in the bloodstream—except tryptophan—begins. Soon thereafter tryptophan enters the brain. Serotonin is synthesized; the stress-regulating system is powered up again, and the unpleasant emotional state you are experiencing begins to dissipate.

You are less angry and upset, more relaxed, and better able to cope. Finally, you no longer feel compelled to eat.

The stress-reducing effects of eating carbohydrates last about three hours. After that, insulin levels decrease with the result that the amino acids that compete with tryptophan for entry to the brain begin to return in the bloodstream, thus allowing less and less tryptophan to get into the brain. Serotonin synthesis slows down and may even cease.

At this point, your unpleasant mood may return, particularly if stress is still present. And your reaction will be familiar: You will again have a craving for carbohydrates. If, on the other hand, the stressful event has passed or, for reasons that we do not understand, your sensitivity to the daily annoyances of life has decreased, then you may not feel the need to consume carbohydrates again.

DISCOVERING CARBOHYDRATE HUNGER: THE RESEARCH

After the connection between eating carbohydrates and increased serotonin production had been established, I became interested in whether rats might have a specific hunger for carbohydrates and whether this hunger might be regulated by serotonin. It seemed reasonable that the brain would make sure it received enough tryptophan to make serotonin by making animals hungry for carbohydrates. After many studies my husband and I were able to publish several papers showing that there really was a specific hunger for carbohydrates in animals. We found that when the animals ate enough carbohydrates to increase serotonin levels in the brain, their appetite for sweet or starchy foods disappeared and they went on to eat other foods, like protein. Later on we treated rats with dexfenfluramine, a drug that was then being used only for research. The drug made serotonin more active.

As a result, the animals lost their appetite for carbohydrate foods and switched to eating protein. This research was the basis for thinking that dexfenfluramine might be able to stop people from bingeing on carbohydrates, too.

Around this time I became interested in studying obesity, in particular why people gain weight after dieting. It was the late 1970s, a period when many obese patients were put on high-protein diets that eliminated all carbohydrate foods. I had the opportunity to work at a local obesity clinic that used such a program and was able to observe what happened to these patients when they returned to normal eating at the end of their diets.

Patient after patient complained about the after-diet inability to stop bingeing, despite extremely careful and compassionate counseling. Two stories of excessive bingeing stand out. In one, a patient told me that while she was doing her weekly food shopping she was overcome by an insatiable need to eat starchy foods. As soon as she got back to the car, she ripped open the wrappings and devoured two loaves of bread.

The other told a poignant tale about visiting his favorite aunt's house a few days before Christmas. There she gave him her yearly gift of a five-pound tin of sugar cookies. On the way home to his wife and children he was seized with such an urge for the cookies that he pulled his car to the side of the road and devoured the entire five pounds.

Why did these people have such an insatiable craving for carbohydrates? I kept thinking about the "carbohydrate hunger" of the rats and I now asked myself several questions. Was there something wrong with the serotonin levels of these bingers? Was it possible that the absence of carbohydrates in their diet program had reduced their serotonin levels? And was this lack leading to uncontrollable eating?

The answer to all three questions was yes.

With the assistance of several colleagues, I now did a study in which rats were put on diets consisting of protein, fat, and fiber—but no carbohydrates. After three weeks, we found that the carbohydrate-deprived rats binged on carbohydrates as soon as they were provided. When we examined the brains of the animals, we found abnormally low amounts of serotonin compared to rats who over the same period of time ate their usual high-carbohydrate rat pellets. No wonder the carbohydrate-deprived rats were bingeing. Their brains were desperate for serotonin.

Did humans binge because of a need for serotonin? It was time to test this theory out on people. We couldn't open up the brains of our human subjects in order to measure serotonin levels, so we needed to find a way to do studies that would give us indirect evidence about the levels of serotonin in individuals who had insatiable appetites for carbohydrates. Borrowing a technique used by researchers who study depression, we designed a study in which people who had intense appetites for carbohydrates would be treated with a drug that increased serotonin activity. If that put an end to the carbohydrate hunger, then we could reasonably assume that serotonin was involved. The drug we used was dexfenfluramine, which by this time had reached the category of a drug that could be tested on people.

When we advertised for volunteers for our study, we were inundated by hundreds of responses from obese men and women who blamed their inability to lose weight on their excess carbohydrate craving. During the initial phase of a series of studies we conducted over the next five years, we asked our volunteers to stay at our Clinical Research Center for periods of several weekends or, in one study, for six weeks. This would enable us to observe their mealtime as well as their snacking food choices.

At mealtimes our dietitians provided a buffet that offered both carbohydrate foods like potatoes, pasta, rice, rolls, stuffing, and muffins, and protein foods such as meat loaf, chicken, tuna salad, eggs, meatballs, seafood salad, and cold cuts. Everything each volunteer chose at each meal was weighed and recorded. We also devised a method for keeping track of snacks. Our volunteers made their selections from a vending machine filled with both protein snacks (like flavored yogurt, cheese, cold cuts, and miniature hot dogs and tiny meatballs) and carbohydrate offerings (like crackers, miniature candy bars, cookies, and chips). Snacks were available twenty-four hours a day, and each volunteer was given a personal access code that activated the machine. A computer hooked up to the machine kept track of who was taking which snacks at what time. Of course, there was no charge for the food. Every day we obtained a computer printout of everything each volunteer ate. Also, we weighed them frequently.

We studied over five hundred people in this manner, and the same thing happened over and over again. At mealtimes there was nothing unusual about the volunteers' selections, nothing to suggest why they were all so overweight or why they craved carbohydrates. They ate a normal mix of carbohydrates and proteins in normal amounts. But snacking was another story. Each day our carbohydrate-craving participants consumed seven hundred to one thousand calories in snacks—none of which was protein. They consistently chose sweet or starchy carbohydrates or a combination of both.

We had expected our overweight volunteers to eat snacks all day. But examination of the computer printouts revealed that each person had a particular time of day, usually two or three hours after lunch or dinner, when he or she would seek out carbohydrates. The rest of the time, very little snacking occurred. Later, we found out that snack times coincided with dramatic changes in mood as well as psychological fatigue. Each person tended to experience a deterioration in their sense of well-being at a specific time, and that was the time at which he or she sought out carbohydrates.

To determine whether inadequate serotonin activity was responsible for the snacking patterns we had observed, we now did a double blind study in which we gave the volunteers, with their consent, either dexfenfluramine or a placebo over a period of several weeks. Not until the end of the study did we or the participants or the nurses who gave them the pills know who was getting what. As we had anticipated, the volunteers on the drug decreased their snack intake substantially—almost by half—while those taking the placebo kept right on eating. This and many other studies like it confirmed our speculation that eating carbohydrates was nature's way of correcting some sort of serotonin imbalance. These studies also yielded additional insight into the connection between snacking behaviors and stress.

The Mood-Food Connection

Our volunteers clued us into the carbohydrate-stress connection. Because they lived at the research center while participating in the study, we had many opportunities to speak with them. I remember one day chatting with a man who ran a travel agency, who was an afternoon snacker. I asked him how he felt before he reached for his snack.

"Distressed and down in the dumps," was his immediate reply. "I can always tell when four o'clock—my snack time—is approaching because I get very down about my business. I hate to make calls to potential clients then because I find it harder to tolerate any negative response to my sales pitch. I start to feel restless and worried. Then something makes me leave my desk and go buy a package of Fig Newtons. What is really interesting is that by the time I eat a couple of cookies, glance at the newspaper, and return to my office, my mood has lifted. I feel more optimistic about work again and more resistant to rejection or lack of interest when I make my calls."

A woman who was an evening snacker and master tournament bridge player told me that when she went to her evening bridge games her handbag was filled with graham crackers.

Around 9 P.M. she would begin to feel the need to eat those crackers. "It didn't matter what I was doing. I became distracted, my attention wandered, and an urge for something sweet took hold. I would excuse myself, find a quiet corner, and eat my crackers. A few minutes later I'd return to the table. After a little while my concentration returned."

At the time I listened to stories like these (about fifteen years ago), the idea that food could affect and alter mood was thought to be absurd. The common explanation for feeling better after eating was that certain foods gave pleasure because of their taste and/or their past associations, or that the very act of taking time off to give yourself a treat was pleasure inducing. So it was with some trepidation that my husband, our colleague Dr. Harris Lieberman, and I set out to see whether carbohydrates might alter mood for biochemical reasons.

By this time we knew that carbohydrates do increase serotonin production and, from studies on depression, that drugs which enhance serotonin's activity do lift people's moods. But whether food-induced changes in serotonin levels and activity could do the same thing as drugs was still to be seen.

We asked obese volunteers who had been staying at our Clinical Research Center to drink two different beverages at different times. One contained enough carbohydrates to boost serotonin levels about ninety minutes after it had been consumed. The other identically tasting beverage contained enough protein to prevent tryptophan from getting into the brain.

Both before consuming the drinks and ninety minutes afterward the volunteers filled out standard psychological tests used to monitor changes in a variety of moods such as anger, energy level, fatigue, calmness, tension, depression, and confusion.

Before consuming either drink the volunteers described themselves as feeling tired and depressed. When the volunteers drank the protein beverage, they experienced no significant change in mood. But when they consumed the carbohydrate-loaded drink they said they felt much better—less depressed and much more energetic. The difference was striking. I remember one volunteer cornering a diet aide and insisting that we had drugged the drink.

He even tried to bribe her into disclosing what was "really in it." Although she repeatedly assured him that the drink contained nothing but carbohydrates, he was incredulous. "I can't believe that I could feel so good after drinking some starch and sugar," he said.

This was a remarkable finding because it enabled us to understand why our volunteers craved carbohydrates when upset. Eating as a reaction to stress could not be explained by self-indulgence, a lack of self-control, or bad habits formed during childhood. In a paper we published about a year after the study, in 1986, we wrote that it seemed as if our volunteers were using carbohydrates as a form of "self-medication." They were trying to restore the brain's stress-management system by ensuring that more serotonin was being made. Something— we still don't understand what—had disturbed the serotonin system so that it was less able to regulate mood, and the brain responded by causing the individual to feel a craving for carbohydrate-rich foods.

The Power of Food

Now that research has shown food can act as a tranquilizer, there has been considerable interest in whether natural foods can be modified to make them better, faster, more effective tranquilizers. Several studies have been done in which different doses and combinations of carbohydrates have been tested to see their effects on making the pattern of amino acids in the blood favorable for tryptophan uptake by the brain.

During the past three years my colleagues and I have been experimenting with carbohydrates that have been altered to enable them to be digested more rapidly and absorbed into the bloodstream more quickly than conventional carbohydrates. We wanted to see if the stress-relief process could be speeded up. One of the substances we have been working on, for example, is a drink specially formulated to counteract some of the changes in mood and appetite that occur in women with PMS.

Although not as potent as the antidepressant drugs that increase serotonin activity, the carbohydrate-based drink boosts serotonin enough to help many women whose PMS is not severe enough to require long-term drug treatment.

Much of the interest in these laboratory-designed foods has been spurred by the food industry, which is beginning to use information from research laboratories to produce a new type of food product called nutraceuticals, or "thera-foods." Nutraceuticals are foods that will not only nourish the body but also enhance chemical processes within the brain that are involved in regulating behavior, mood, memory, and alertness. Nutraceuticals, like the food substances my colleagues and I have been working on, are altered so that they quickly enter the bloodstream and powerfully affect brain chemistry. With no protein to slow down tryptophan's entry into the brain, and no fat to add empty calories, these scientifically designed carbohydrates act like potatoes or pasta on the chemistry of the brain—only faster and more efficiently. Nutraceuticals are not limited to carbohydrate combinations. Some contain purified substances from eggs or soybeans that might have an impact on preventing memory loss; others contain amino acids thought to help in promoting mental alertness.

Obviously, people with serious mood disorders like clinical depression or other kinds of mental problems should not depend on either foods or nutraceuticals to make them feel better. A medical problem requires a medical solution. For example, women with severe PMS will probably find more relief from psychoactive drugs than from food. However, it is reasonable to expect that in the near future serotonin-boosting foods or food products could be combined effectively with psychoactive drugs. When this happens, the food plans in this book may be able to play a role as one element in a medically prescribed treatment plan—for example, for clinical depression.

For those of us who simply suffer from the stresses of everyday life, the mood changes brought on by monthly hormonal fluctuations, the down-in-the-dumps gloom brought on by dark winter days, and other relatively routine problems like after-diet food cravings and those that ex-smokers face, no drugs are necessary. We can relieve our stresses naturally, with food, and we can start doing it now. The key is not avoiding sweet or starchy carbohydrates but choosing the right ones.

LET THEM EAT CAKE, NOT STEAK— OR STRAWBERRIES

It is important to recognize that serotonin hunger can be satisfied *only* by eating carbohydrates. Our carbohydrate-craving volunteers knew this intuitively, consistently rejecting the vending machine's protein snacks in favor of the sweet and starchy ones. But many of you who are trying to lose weight have been so brainwashed by the various diet programs you've followed that you fully believe carbohydrates spell doom to your efforts. So, even when protein is unappealing, you reach for it, or for fruit, in an effort to stave off a binge but end up with a brain that is still desperately seeking serotonin.

Tom is an example of someone who ignored his brain's signals. Whenever work made him upset and agitated he would leave his office and go to a nearby fast-food restaurant, where he would eat six or seven large hamburgers at one sitting.

When he told me this I assumed he craved protein—a common phenomenon in certain dieters—and that he probably threw away the hamburger rolls. I was surprised when he explained that he not only didn't throw them away—he considered them the best part of the meal. He ate the burgers first and saved the best part for last: the rolls soaked with pickle and hamburger juice.

Upon further questioning I found out that he had been on an extremely low-carbohydrate diet and had convinced himself that he wanted meat when he started bingeing because it made him feel less guilty. But when he admitted that the only part of the meal he really craved was the buns, it was clear to me that brain chemistry is stronger than any brainwashing that says carbohydrates are taboo.

Fruits are the only carbohydrate foods that do not relieve stress. While fruits are a wonderful-tasting source of vitamins, minerals, and fiber and should be part of everyone's diet, they don't provide the serotonin boost of other carbohydrates (see page 21). If you have ever noticed that you still feel psychologically hungry after eating fruit, this is the reason.

Not by Bread Alone

It may seem that I'm telling you protein is now to be considered "bad," while carbohydrates are "good." Nothing could be further from the truth. Protein—poultry, fish, red meat, dairy products, eggs, and soy products—is essential to life. Protein supplies certain amino acids that our bodies do not manufacture, and protein-rich foods also contain important vitamins and minerals.

You must supply your body with protein. The problem is this: How can you get the protein you need for health without interfering with the serotonin production required for emotional well-being and appetite control? How can proteins and carbohydrates both do their jobs without the former undermining the latter?

It's not easy. Every time you eat protein, you elevate the concentrations of the amino acids that compete with tryptophan for as long as three hours after digestion. This means that if you eat a three- to four-ounce turkey or tuna sandwich at noon, the amino acids from the poultry or fish will remain in your blood until three or four in the afternoon, inhibiting tryptophan from entering the brain.

Fortunately, my colleagues and I have discovered in our research the exact amount of protein that can be consumed with carbohydrates without causing a buildup of amino acids in the blood. The ratio is one part protein to five parts carbohydrates. For instance, if you eat one ounce of turkey, eat five ounces of stuffing along with it; eat one meatball for five ounces of spaghetti; just moisten your breakfast cereal with milk, rather than immersing it.

All of the food plans in this book are based on what we know about how different combinations of protein and carbohydrates affect biochemical processes in the blood and the brain, and how long these effects last. When you read through the individual food plans, you'll notice that some meals contain much more protein than others, and for a very good reason. It's because there are certain times of day when you are less likely to need the stress-relieving effects of carbohydrates, and you can use these periods to meet your daily protein requirements. Follow these food plans exactly to get maximum value from both your protein and carbohydrate consumption. When and in what combination you eat these foods is as important as how much of them you eat, because all the recommendations are based on overall considerations of health in combination with a scientific analysis of how easy or hard it will be for tryptophan to enter the brain after any particular meal or snack is eaten.

GREASING THE BINGE: WHY YOU SHOULD AVOID FAT-FILLED FOODS

Unfortunately, most of the sweet or starchy foods we reach for when we are experiencing emotional distress—potato chips, ice cream, buttery cookies, or chocolate—also contain a lot of fat. We tend to eat them very quickly and in large amounts because they taste so good and because they're "forbidden." When we feel in dire need of comfort, we say to ourselves, "Life has been lousy to me today. I deserve something special. I don't care if it packs a zillion calories; I *need* it to make me feel good." Unfortunately, these treats *don't* make us feel good. Even though they contain lots of carbohydrates, you don't get the calmness or comfort that I've described as the outcome of serotonin production. Instead, you feel lethargic, slowed down, almost zombielike.

The reason this is so is that large quantities of fatty foods seem to interfere with the workings of the stress-management system. A brain chemical called galanin, which is activated by fat consumption, competes with serotonin and overwhelms it. When too much galanin is made, according to Dr. Sara Leibowitz, a professor at Rockefeller University who identified this chemical, people feel passive and tired, unable to think clearly. This, combined with the fact that fat takes a long time to be digested, means that the effects of a high-fat meal or snack can last for hours, which is why so many people end up simply going to sleep after a high-fat dinner.

Fat as a Feeling Blocker

Carol had an experience many of us can relate to: At a meeting at work she had had to watch her boss make a presentation based on her ideas, and then take credit for them himself. Although it was excruciating to remain silent, she did—neither the time nor the place was right for a confrontation. Too agitated to return to her office right away, she left the scene as soon as she could, ostensibly to cool off. Instead, she found herself in the lobby snack shop, surrounded by boxes of candy on display for next week's holiday, Mother's Day. "Chocolate. *That's* what I want," she thought to herself, buying a two-pound box. As soon as she was back in her locked office, she tore it open and dug in. Twenty minutes later the box was empty.

When Carol told me this story two weeks after it happened, she was still upset. She told me, with a look of disbelief on her face, that at the rate she'd been going nothing would have made her stop eating the candy unless someone had knocked on the door. "How could I possibly have eaten the whole box?" she asked. "Especially since chocolate has so much fat in it that you'd think I would have felt sated long before finishing. But I didn't even feel full after I ate every piece. I think if I had bought another box, I would have eaten that, too."

When I asked her how she felt an hour and a half later, she grimaced and told me she'd felt numb. "My rage and agitation had disappeared by then. But they seemed to be replaced by a dullness, an almost total lack of feeling. I sat at my desk, but work was out of the question. My head felt too fuzzy."

Many people binge on fat-laden carbohydrates not just for their taste but because they want to *sustain* the emotion-blocking effects of fat. They don't want the calm feelings and improved coping ability, which is one of the major effects of serotonin. They want to *smother* their emotions. And that's what happens with fat. If you eat enough fat-filled foods, you become passive and unresponsive: The muddled, tired, stuffed feeling they create won't allow you to feel anything.

Mary, a client of mine whose husband was dying of cancer, told me the only way she could maintain her composure sitting by his bed was to fill herself up with fatty foods every two or three hours. At the hospital cafeteria she ate fried foods, mashed potatoes with gravy, lots of butter, and rich desserts. Thus "anesthetized," she could resume her bedside vigil.

Jane, an overweight young woman who had a lifelong struggle with her weight, is another example. When she came to see me, she had recently broken off a long relationship and found herself facing the summer alone; she was worried about the impact it might have on her diet. Weekdays, she said, weren't too difficult. She was kept busy at her job as an advertising copywriter and didn't allow herself to feel the sadness that might have led to binge eating. Friday nights and Saturdays weren't too bad either. She spent the weekends in a beach house she shared with friends where her eating remained under control. Sunday night, however, was a different story.

On her way home on Sunday afternoon, she would always stop at a roadside stand to have a large plate of fried clams with tartar sauce, French fries, and mayonnaise-drenched coleslaw. Dessert was a slice of blueberry pie topped with vanilla ice cream. Once back in the city, she would buy a tuna sub and potato chips to eat at the Laundromat while doing the week's laundry. On the way back to her apartment, she would have an ice cream cone.

Home again, she tried to get ready for the week ahead but found herself so tired and lethargic that she ended up lying on the couch, trying to read but instead watching television until she fell asleep.

"Why are you eating this way?" I asked her each time she recited these Sunday menus.

"I love those foods," she replied testily. "Why shouldn't I eat what I like?"

I agreed with her that most people would like those foods and that indeed everyone should eat what they want. "But why sabotage your diet so deliberately every week? What is it about Sunday?"

Finally she admitted that driving home she felt the pain of the transition from a carefree weekend with friends to another week of loneliness without her boyfriend. She couldn't stand coming home to an empty apartment.

"I guess I use food to dull my pain," she said. "The closer I get to home the more depressed and agitated I become. I know if I followed your suggestion to eat something sweet or starchy without much fat I would feel better. But I just don't want to feel anything. I don't want to think of what I have to do for the week ahead. I don't want to feel responsible for my apartment or checking account or try to make plans to reactivate my social life. The food makes me tired and numb, which is what I want."

The Less Fat the Better

In addition to activating galanin, fat interferes with the brain's stress-management system in another important way. Fat does not enter the bloodstream as quickly as either protein or carbohydrate, because fat takes longer to digest. It may take as long as two or three hours for fat to be digested and enter the bloodstream along with the carbohydrates that will stimulate serotonin. After a high-fat snack like ice cream or cheesecake your brain doesn't receive the signal to tell you to slow down and stop; in the meantime you just keep eating. But by that point, you are likely to have consumed an enormous number of calories and grams of fat. And you feel awful.

Now think about what happens when you substitute fat-free cookies, for example, for the fat-filled snacks. As soon as you swallow them, your body begins to process them. Within minutes, the first small amounts of digested carbohydrates begin to enter your bloodstream. In about thirty minutes, serotonin has begun to exert its braking effect on your appetite. You start to feel full; the agitation that is driving you to eat lessens, and soon thereafter you stop eating. And you feel content.

Fat and Eating Control

Small amounts of fat are necessary in our diets because fat provides essential nutrients such as fatty acids and vitamins E and A. As you will see in later chapters, all of the food plans include one to two fat servings every day. If you are following a plan to maintain, not lose, weight, then you can increase your calories by adding one or two more fat exchanges to your daily intake.

Make sure, however, that the carbohydrate snack foods you eat to maintain serotonin levels remain as fat free as possible. There are several benefits to doing this. Keeping fat to a minimum means keeping calories low as well. Fat contains more than twice as many calories per gram as carbohydrates—nine calories a gram for fat, versus four calories a gram for carbohydrates. Since you are allocated approximately two hundred calories for a snack (see Chapter Five), if you reduce the amount of fat you eat you'll be able to have a larger serving of carbohydrates. And, of course, less fat means a more immediate sensation of relief.

Fortunately, there is now a wide variety of low- or fat-free foods available—including cakes, cookies, and ice creams—that have been formulated to duplicate the taste of butter or cream. Many taste quite delicious and impart the sensual pleasure we seek. And they provide the subsequent emotional relief without interference from the brain chemical galanin.

But following the guidelines to decrease or avoid fat in your diet does not mean that you can never again indulge in a wickedly rich dessert. Of course there should be occasions when we allow ourselves to enjoy a favorite food even if its fat content equals a week's quota. But these foods should be regarded as special, not typical, for celebrations only! It comes down to this: Routinely eating high-fat foods cannot be justified. A diet in which no more than 20 percent of the calories come from fat is the widely accepted standard for maintaining general health. Even if fat were not associated with such medical problems as heart disease and diabetes, its effect on subverting the serotonin stress-relief system is enough reason to avoid it as much as possible.

If you still feel tempted to binge on high-fat foods when you are distressed, ask yourself how you want to feel an hour or two later. The choice is between comatose and calm, inert and alert. One mode allows you to escape your problems, the other to confront them. Don't smother your coping system with fat.

HOW MUCH CARBOHYDRATE IS ENOUGH?

After years of research, we have discovered that for most people under normal amounts of stress, about forty grams of carbohydrate (about one and a half ounces)—the amount contained in one regular size bagel, six graham crackers, one cup of pasta, or a small potato—is enough to produce the serotonin surge they need to get mood and appetite under control. And although fresh bagels and potatoes don't come with labels, just about everything else does. If you are unsure about how much carbohydrate a serving of your favorite sweet or starchy snack contains, just read the label on the package. In Chapter Five you will receive a brief course in label reading so you can figure out whether you are getting as much carbohydrate as you should be.

TIMED RELIEF

Once you've dosed yourself with the carbohydrate of your choice, you must wait a brief period before you can expect to feel the benefits. As you understand by now, the necessary changes in the brain do not occur immediately after you eat a sweet or starchy food. It takes about thirty minutes for the soothing effect of serotonin to kick in. If your stomach was completely empty it might take less time, and if you eat the snack while still digesting food from a previous meal or snack, the effect may be delayed an additional ten to fifteen minutes. Stress relief is gradual, sort of like taking pain medication for a headache. After all, you don't expect your headache to be gone seconds after swallowing pain medication. In fact, you often don't feel any change for fifteen minutes after taking the pill and may not even be aware that the headache is entirely gone for another fifteen minutes or even longer. However, once the pain begins to recede you may find yourself going about your business without even remembering the previous discomfort. The same gradual improvement in mood occurs after eating carbohydrates. Sometimes you don't even register the change unless someone asks how you are feeling. The calmness and comfort you will experience lasts about three hours.

Remember: Never continue to eat until you feel better. If you still don't feel any improvement after thirty to forty minutes, you can eat more then. But chances are that if you wait, you will lose your interest and your need to eat.

I have seen this happen in volunteers who drank carbohydrate-rich beverages at certain times of day to see how the drinks affected their stress levels and appetite. They were certain they would want to eat after finishing the drink. But they found to their surprise that after thirty to forty minutes had passed, they were no longer searching for something to eat. Since the experimental drink contained under two hundred calories, it wasn't the calories that were filling them up. Rather, it was the carbohydrate acting on their serotonin systems that was shutting off their appetites.

CHAPTER THREE

The Diet Wreckers: Recognizing Situational and Biological Stress

There are two basic kinds of stress that result in the carbohydrate-craving serotonin-seeking eating behavior I've been discussing: situational stress—that is, stress stemming from events outside the body—and biological stress, which is built into our bodily systems. But *both* have a biochemical effect on serotonin. The first kind of stress includes any of the annoyances, minor and major, that happen to us daily. The stress of being a full-time mommy and daily stress fall into the situational stress category. Those of us vulnerable to this kind of stress find that as the difficulties of the day pile up, we become less and less able to cope or to filter out worries or deal with anger and tension. For reasons not fully understood, the serotonin that fuels our stress-management system has been depleted or rendered less effective.

The other kind of stress is triggered by biological events within the body over which we have no control. While some of these biological stressors may have a negative impact on our mood, they are conditions that either directly or indirectly affect the serotonin stress-management system regardless of our state of mind. Included in this category are premenstrual syndrome, seasonal affective disorder (also known as winter depression), smoking withdrawal, and shift work. These stressors cause the same kinds of problems as situational stress. Why some people are vulnerable to these stressors and other people are not we don't yet know. But we have learned a lot about how to use carbohydrates in carefully timed and measured doses to relieve the various stresses that fall into either of these categories.

DAILY STRESS

Most of us have a daily rhythm that governs our moods, our ability to cope, and our eating patterns. It causes us, almost instinctively, to work harder at certain times of day, to be more cheerful or grumpy according to an internal clock, to move slowly or quickly, to be relaxed or nervous, to have control over our eating or to give way to cravings and binges. We don't know why it exists, but it does.

One of the key variables in this daily rhythm is the degree to which we are able to handle stress. Many of us seem to lose this capacity at certain times. We overreact to problems, find it hard to focus on work, and feel tired even if we've done no more than sit in front of the TV all day. An argument we deflect with humor at one time of day becomes a lengthy quarrel at another.

The serotonin-seeker's diet plan in Chapter Five is designed to meet the needs of those who overeat because of daily stress. It ensures that you will never have to choose between giving in to stress-driven cravings and trying to bear the emotional distress of your day without relief. The plan provides a food prescription for coping. It will control your eating and help you reach your diet goals. Moreover, once you meet your weight-loss goals, you can adapt the plan to weight maintenance by simply adding extra calories but eating the same ratio of carbohydrates to proteins. You can use the plan as a lifelong way to keep your serotonin stress-management system in good working order.

MOMMY STRESS

Full-time moms with stay-at-home kids are vulnerable to a particular type of stressful overeating. Erratic feeding schedules, unending fatigue, unexpected bouts of illness, bad weather that keeps you and the kids housebound, and the squabbling, the messes, and the loneliness—these can trigger eating. And although the children will become toilet trained, grow up, and increase their culinary choices beyond Cheerios and apple juice, for the mother at home alone this is sometimes hard—if not impossible—to believe.

Although stretch pants may be one answer to the weight gained by stressed mommies who stay at home with preschool children, the stressed-mommy diet is the better solution.

This diet is designed to compensate for the enormous demands exacted on the serotonin stress-management system by a mother's need to stay cool, patient, and reasonable, hour after hour. As serotonin stores are depleted by the never-ending chain of daily irritants, the stay-at-home mom responds by eating, often. Then after a day of nibbling on your children's leftovers—soggy bread crusts, cold French fries, the dregs of a glass of chocolate milk, a half-filled box of animal crackers—you usually have to prepare and eat dinner. Sometimes twice. There's the five to six o'clock meal you make for the kids, then the one you eat later with your partner.

The stressed-mommy diet (see Chapter Six) gives you an eating plan timed to the special rhythms of your day. Its daytime high-carbohydrate content will keep serotonin levels elevated when you need them to be, while at night, when the children are asleep and your serotonin system is not so stressed, the dinner choices give you the protein necessary for good health. This plan is not only for full-time mothers. It is recommended for working mothers on weekends and vacations and for anyone—dads and grandparents included—who takes care of preschool children.

PREMENSTRUAL STRESS

Changes in mood, appetite, concentration, memory, and physical well-being occur predictably in many women during the last week or so of their menstrual cycles as a result of premenstrual stress (PMS). The number of symptoms associated with PMS have been estimated by Dr. Uriel Halbreich of the University of Buffalo Medical School to be as high as two hundred.

One of the most annoying manifestations of PMS is a significant increase in appetite, especially for sweet and starchy foods. Even the strictest calorie counter can find herself devouring a large portion of something fattening during this time of the month. I have a close friend who normally watches every morsel of food she eats. Her kitchen is a fat-free zone; her idea of a treat is a bowl of cereal with skim milk.

A few months ago we spent a day doing errands and browsing in some rarely visited city neighborhoods. At one point during our walk we passed a bakery. "I have to go in," my friend declared, leaving me on the sidewalk as she raced inside. Following her, I saw that she was pointing to a large chocolate-frosted brownie. "Don't bother to wrap it," she instructed the clerk as she paid her bill.

A few minutes later the brownie was gone.

"PMS?" I asked.

"Of course," she replied.

No one knows exactly how many women suffer from PMS; estimates range from 4 to 30 percent of the female population. Nor is it understood why some women are affected with PMS each month, while others rarely or never experience its symptoms. In fact, the questions about PMS outweigh the answers.

But what is known now is that the monthly changes in hormone levels alter (in ways not yet understood) the neurotransmitter systems in the brain. As a result, serotonin appears to become less effective at stress and appetite control. Recent reports have suggested that women with PMS who suffer debilitating changes in mood can be helped by the antidepressant drug Prozac, because of its role in restoring serotonin activity to normal. Other medications, such as Zoloft and Paxil, are also now being tested for use in alleviating PMS. It is even possible that the weight-loss drug dexfenfluramine (Redux) may eventually be used as well. Dr. Amnon Brzenzinski of Hebrew University/Hadassah Medical School and I have done studies to show that Redux works both to diminish premenstrual depression and to curb excessive appetite.

However, for most women with PMS the use of drug therapy month after month is not an option. If their symptoms aren't severe enough to justify drug therapy, or they don't want to take drugs that might affect them if they become pregnant, the premenstrual stress diet may be just what they need. While no food can act in the body with the intensity of medication, for most women this food plan will do an excellent job of renewing and restoring serotonin activity, while also enabling them to halt impulsive overeating and thus lose weight.

The mind-over-menstrual-cycle diet (see Chapter Seven) comes in plain and chocolate-coated versions. Either way, it provides frequent, tasty doses of carbohydrates. So not only will your premenstrual taste buds rejoice but also your premenstrual serotonin will function optimally.

Since each woman's experience of PMS is unique, you must be the judge of when the symptoms you are experiencing—especially a lack of eating control—call for frequent therapeutic doses of carbohydrates. You may want to follow the plan for six or seven days—or six or seven hours. Use the diet plan as needed. When your PMS is over, switch back to the serotonin-seeker's diet. If weight loss is not your goal but you're concerned about premenstrual stress and out-of-control eating, follow the general principles of the PMS plan but add 400 to 600 extra calories to each day's quota.

SHIFT-WORK STRESS

Body clocks that are tampered with trigger overeating. Whether you are a medical resident, television reporter, or factory worker, if you work a night shift you are all too familiar with the weight gain that comes from changing your body clock. You know the drill. On workdays you must get up and go to bed according to your work schedule, but on your days off you return to the world of daytime wakefulness and nighttime sleep, even though this might be the exact opposite of your work routine. And this alteration may take place every six or seven days.

Waking up when your internal clock is directing you to sleep and forcing yourself to sleep when that same clock is sounding a wake-up alarm has two results: chronic stress and overeating. I first became aware of the steep price paid in pounds by shift-workers when I was giving continuing education classes to nurses. They told me they overate to stay awake and also to get themselves to sleep. Many claimed that gaining twenty pounds in a year was not unusual.

Ironically, using food as a tool to keep the body awake and quiet it down for sleep is instinctively correct. The problem is that most people who use food for these purposes don't know how to do it effectively. And instead of causing wakefulness or sleepiness at the appropriate times, the food ends up causing weight gain.

As you will see in Chapter Nine, the shift-work diet also takes into account the particular stresses and dilemmas of a night owl existence in order to solve the eating problems that typically accompany that lifestyle. The diet is carefully planned to take advantage of current research findings on the effects of food on both wakefulness and sleepiness. You will be able to lose weight while simultaneously resetting your body clock.

SEASONAL AFFECTIVE DISORDER (SAD) STRESS

You may not be aware that the reason you always gain weight in the winter and lose it in the summer is due to a seasonally induced fluctuation in mood and appetite. Perhaps you have assumed you eat more in the winter to keep warm and eat less in the summer because it's too hot. It's not as simple as that.

Unless you live on the equator, where the hours of daylight and darkness are constant year-round, the change of seasons affects the length of the daylight hours. The further north or south of the equator you live, the more noticeable these changes are.

It has been discovered that the seasonal changes in the amount of daylight may have an effect on our brains, thereby altering our feelings of sleepiness and alertness, calmness and irritability, apathy and enthusiasm, and fatigue and vigor. These same seasonal changes may have a drastic effect on appetite as well. It is not unusual for some people to develop a ravenous appetite that persists throughout the fall and winter. Studies carried out by Dr. Norman Rosenthal and his colleagues at the National Institute of Mental Health show that weight gains of as much as forty pounds in a season are not uncommon. Dr. Rosenthal coined the term "seasonal affective disorder" to describe this condition. Rosenthal and others working on the disorder also found that people who suffered from it exhibited an uncontrollable craving for sweet or starchy foods.

A loss of appetite, especially for carbohydrates, may mark the other side of the seasonal pendulum. Those who gain weight during the darkness of winter are often able to lose pounds during the long hours of daylight during the summer.

Serotonin is implicated in these seasonal changes. Working with Dr. Dermot O'Rourke, a research and practicing psychiatrist, during the course of three consecutive falls and winters, I conducted studies on the role of serotonin in the mood and appetite changes of seasonal affective disorder. Our research showed that when patients suffering from SAD were treated with dexfenfluramine, they ate less and lost weight, and their moods returned to normal. Subsequently, others who have used antidepressant drugs like Prozac, which work to increase serotonin activity in a fashion similar to dexfenfluramine, confirm the role of serotonin in this disorder and the usefulness of drug or food therapies that spur serotonin production.

I have developed the two-part seasonally adjusted diet to suit the special needs of those who experience seasonal fluctuations in appetite and weight (and often in mood as well). During the fall and winter, when your appetite is at its height, you will follow a high-carbohydrate diet designed to minimize weight gain. When your appetite decreases in the spring and summer, you will follow a diet designed for rapid weight loss. Even though half the year will be spent in preventing weight gain, the weight loss you will achieve with the spring-summer diet will allow you to finish the year thinner than when it began.

Begin the winter phase of the diet by mid-to-late-fall, when you first notice increased fatigue, sagging spirits, and the pointer on the scale inching upward. By late spring, when you are energized by the long daylight hours and feel an overwhelming sense of well-being, you should begin the spring/summer quick weight-loss plan. Pounds will come off easily until the leaves start to change color and the days become noticeably shorter. At that point, go back to the winter diet plan.

EX-SMOKER STRESS

For most smokers, weight gain goes hand in hand with giving up cigarettes. The out-of-control eating that so often occurs in ex-smokers is not just the urge to put something in the mouth as a cigarette substitute; it is a response to nicotine withdrawal. As you will read in Chapter Ten, nicotine is a powerful drug with powerful effects on the brain. When it is suddenly absent, the brain has a lot of readjusting to do.

One of the brain functions affected by both the presence and absence of nicotine is the serotonin stress-management system. Nicotine acts on some of the same brain systems as does serotonin. When a person stops smoking, the brain reacts as if not enough serotonin is present. The result is mood changes, insomnia, inability to concentrate, and fatigue—all the signs of inadequate serotonin function. In order to keep everything working normally, the brain demands extra amounts of serotonin. Hence the constant need to eat sweet or starchy carbohydrates.

I have developed the ex-smoker's stress plan to deal with these problems. It is not, however, a weight-loss plan, because trying to diet and give up smoking simultaneously is doomed to failure. The brain simply won't allow the ex-smoker to deprive it of both nicotine and food at the same time. Though weight loss is impossible under the circumstances, you can *prevent* weight gain by using my plan to get you through the first weeks without cigarettes. As the food plans renew and restore serotonin levels, you will find yourself able to withstand the feeling of deprivation caused by lack of nicotine. Your sleep patterns will improve. And, best of all, your cravings and appetite will again be under control. At that point you can, if you choose, decide to go on one of the serotonin-enhancing weight-loss plans in the book. Your body will be ready.

AFTER-DIET STRESS

The after-diet binge phenomenon is so prevalent that it accounts for countless long-term memberships in the weight-loss programs that are flourishing today. Who can forget the Oprah Winfrey Optifast debacle? As Winfrey herself has since shown, this does not have to happen if you follow a sensible diet that contains sufficient carbohydrates.

For the rest of us I have devised a brief (only a week long) food plan that will ease you into a maintenance eating program without the risk of your eating spinning out of control. As you will see in Chapter Eleven, the diet is particularly useful if you are coming off a low-calorie liquid meal replacement plan or one of the newly fashionable low-carbohydrate diet plans, or weaning yourself from a weight-loss support group.

When I learned of research in England that showed significant changes in brain serotonin after dieters spent only three weeks on a relatively low-carbohydrate diet, I understood why so many of our subjects began to gain weight within two weeks of ending a diet. It was not because maintenance techniques weren't working. It was because their serotonin control systems weren't functioning.

Follow the after-diet eating plan if you have been on a

carbohydrate-deficient diet. After completing the week's plan, go on to the basic serotonin-seeker's diet plan or other relevant plan.

If you recognize yourself in any of the stress situations or the eating behaviors described in this chapter, you can use *The Serotonin Solution* to make sure your serotonin stress-management system will always be functional, regardless of the problems you are facing. The seven different food plans in the book each prescribe the correct timing and "doses" for carbohydrate relief from your particular kind of stress. All you have to do is this: Understand what the various stress triggers are (see Chapter Four), whether or not you are affected by them, and which food plans to choose. The plans have an extra benefit: They will allow you to either lose weight or maintain it, depending on your needs at any given time.

CHAPTER FOUR

The Questionnaires, or, "Know Thyself"

KNOW YOUR TRIGGERS

Unless you understand what makes you overeat, you will be doomed to keep regaining the weight you lose. Unfortunately, if you have lost weight on an organized weight-loss program, you are never questioned as to why you regained your weight when you sign up again. This is true despite the incredibly high rate of recidivism among participants of diet programs—at least 70 percent of all Weight Watchers members are repeat dieters, according to a report issued by the National Task Force on the Prevention and Treatment of Obesity.

The assumption instead is that it's your fault. *If* you had really learned how to incorporate a healthy eating style into your life and *if* you had been really committed to exercising, then you wouldn't be signing up for yet another round of classes.

Years ago I questioned a member of the corporate board of a national diet program on its approach to yo-yo dieting—as constant weight gain and loss is sometimes called. The director calmly assured me that because the program was so well designed, few, if any, participants regained their lost weight. I was invited to attend a few maintenance sessions so that I could see for myself how effective their program was.

I arrived at the weight-loss facility early and found the reception area filled to capacity with about fifty people, all of whom were overweight. I assumed they were part of an ongoing weight-loss program, since it was obvious that none had reached a target weight. However, I was surprised by the conversations I overheard, which were the kind typical of people who hadn't seen each other in a long time—not of people who were accustomed to getting together weekly. "How has your year gone?" "Is the new job still working out?" "Did you ever get to move into that new apartment?"

And indeed when I asked one of the participants about the gathering, it turned out everyone in the room had completed the weight-loss program some ten months earlier. This was their first reunion since then. "We're all here because we're starting a special program designed for past participants who have regained the weight they lost last year," the woman explained.

"Oh," I said, trying to sound innocent, "I thought no one regained weight after going through maintenance."

She gave me a look that spoke volumes as she turned away to greet another formerly thin friend.

Since the causes of overeating reside in the chemistry of the brain, we are always tempted to eat too much when our emotional well-being is challenged. Unfortunately, losing weight does not change your vulnerability to stress-driven overeating. The only way to change this pattern is to learn to recognize the kinds of stress that create a drain on the serotonin eating-control system. Once you can identify your stress triggers, you can choose the appropriate food plan in the book to prevent your serotonin system from becoming depleted.

THE OVEREATING SELF-ASSESSMENT TESTS

Following are a series of questionnaires designed to determine which overeating triggers are most responsible for *your* weight gain. Take your time with these tests; you may not have noticed how automatically your eating patterns respond to some of the triggers described in these lists, and several of them may take a while to become apparent. For example, if these questionnaires now prompt you to wonder if your eating changes when you are premenstrual or with the onset of winter, then wait until the appropriate time to answer the questions that deal with those particular triggers.

Daily Stress Questionnaire

1. Which of the four eating patterns below resembles the way you eat?

> a. three meals a day and rarely eat between meals or after the evening meal
> b. three meals a day and one or more between-meals or after-meal snack
> c. do not start eating until late afternoon and dinner and then eat until you go to sleep
> d. nibble all day and rarely eat meals

If you answered *a*, it is unlikely that you are eating too much because of stress.

If you answered *c*, you may or may not be eating too much from stress. You could also be eating too much because you have no idea of how much you are ingesting. Put yourself on three meals a day and then see what happens. And answer the rest of the questionnaire.

If you answered *b* or *d*, it suggests that your snacking is a daily stress-driven activity. The basic serotonin-seeker's diet will be perfect for you because it allows you to snack every day. When you eat your high-carbohydrate low-fat snack should correspond to the time you currently eat your between-meals snack.

2. What do you prefer snacking on? (Be completely honest. Do not avoid the high-calorie answers.) Circle the items that apply.

A	B	C
raw vegetables	nuts	crackers
fruit	peanut butter	cookies
yogurt	bacon	tortilla chips
cottage cheese	cheese	popcorn
tuna	pork rinds	bagels
milk		muffins
hamburger		doughnuts
soup		candy
beef jerky		ice cream
leftover meat or chicken		frozen yogurt
cold cuts		pizza
		cold cereal

If most of your choices came from column C, then you are a serotonin-seeking stress snacker, deliberately seeking out carbohydrate foods. If you occasionally chose fruit, yogurt, or leftover meat (from column A) or once in a while grab a handful of nuts or a slice of cheese (from column B), you still fit the stress-snacker profile.

But if most of the items you circled were protein foods, fruits, and vegetables from column A, or the high-fat low-carbohydrate foods from column B, you are not a stress-driven snacker. You may simply snack out of boredom or habit as opposed to eating to make yourself feel better. You may still benefit from this plan, however. It will teach you to select comforting, less fattening foods, regardless of whether your drive to eat is caused by stress, boredom, or habit.

Answer the following questions using the scale of 1 to 10, 1 being rarely and 10 being always or very often.

3. How often do you snack when you are upset or stressed?
   1   2   3   4   5   6   7   8   9   10

4. Does your eating go out of control when you are stressed?
   1   2   3   4   5   6   7   8   9   10

5. How often do you go off a diet when you are stressed?

    1   2   3   4   5   6   7   8   9   10

6. How often do you experience uncontrollable urges for sweet and starchy foods when you are stressed?

    1   2   3   4   5   6   7   8   9   10

If you answered all these questions with the number 6 or above, then you are almost surely a stress-driven snacker who would do well on the basic serotonin-seeker's diet.

The Stressed-Mommy Questionnaire

Stay-at-home mommies with small children have their own set of special stresses. Answer the following questions to see if you experience any of these triggers.

1. Do you find that you eat all day but can't remember anything you put in your mouth?

2. Is your house filled with tempting snack foods you bought for your children but can't keep from eating yourself?

3. Is your ability to control your eating eroded by the need to spend hours preparing foods, feeding your children, and cleaning up after them, over and over again?

4. Do you eat to keep yourself going after being up all night with a crying baby?

5. Do you eat to give yourself a break from an afternoon with a whiny toddler?

6. Do you eat to prevent yourself from screaming at fighting siblings?

7. Do you ever actually sit down to eat during the day?

8. Are your daytime menu selections limited to foods that can be chewed without teeth?

If you have replied yes to any of these queries (except number 7), read Chapter Six and follow the stressed-mommy diet. It is designed to aid you, the woman at home with young children, in controlling the overeating that comes with the territory. Unlike other food plans in this book, this one is compatible with the unique lifestyle of a stay-at-home caretaker with preschool kids. Although it is meant to be followed daily by those at home all the time, it can certainly be used by anyone who works outside the home and then returns to the second job of child care on weekends and days off.

Premenstrual Syndrome Questionnaire

If you are not sure whether you experience PMS, use the questionnaire below to find out. Those of you who have not noticed any connection between your monthly hormonal fluctuations and your mood and appetite should use the questionnaire during three consecutive cycles, paying particular attention to the second half of each cycle. This will help you determine whether your mood and appetite changes are random or cyclical in nature.

Circle the appropriate number for each symptom: 0 = none, 1 = mild, 2 = moderate, 3 = severe.

SYMPTOMS	WEEK BEFORE PERIOD	WEEK AFTER PERIOD
tension	0 1 2 3	0 1 2 3
irritability	0 1 2 3	0 1 2 3
mood out of control	0 1 2 3	0 1 2 3
anxiety	0 1 2 3	0 1 2 3
difficulty concentrating	0 1 2 3	0 1 2 3
anger	0 1 2 3	0 1 2 3
depression	0 1 2 3	0 1 2 3
exhaustion	0 1 2 3	0 1 2 3
confusion	0 1 2 3	0 1 2 3
clumsiness	0 1 2 3	0 1 2 3
forgetfulness	0 1 2 3	0 1 2 3
impaired work ability	0 1 2 3	0 1 2 3
cravings for sweet or starchy foods	0 1 2 3	0 1 2 3
cravings for salty foods	0 1 2 3	0 1 2 3

SYMPTOMS	WEEK BEFORE PERIOD	WEEK AFTER PERIOD
hunger	0 1 2 3	0 1 2 3
sleep disturbances	0 1 2 3	0 1 2 3

Look at how you answered each item. If you have PMS, then your scores before your period should be higher than your scores after it for at least four to six items. Your scores on the others can be the same for both weeks. However, if your scores for the week after your period are higher than those of the week before it (for at least four to six items), then you definitely don't have PMS.

The table below provides the sample answer of a woman who is suffering from the mood swings and overeating typical of PMS.

SYMPTOMS	WEEK BEFORE PERIOD	WEEK AFTER PERIOD
tension	3	1
irritability	3	0
mood out of control	2	0
anxiety	3	2
difficulty concentrating	3	0
anger	2	1
depression	2	0
exhaustion	3	1
confusion	2	1
clumsiness	2	0
forgetfulness	3	2
impaired work ability	3	0
cravings for sweet or starchy foods	3	2
cravings for salty foods	1	0
hunger	1	0
sleep disturbances	2	0

Seasonal Weight Change Questionnaire

If you have never paid attention to your seasonal weight gain and loss patterns, ask yourself if your winter clothes are a size larger than your summer outfits. Consider how often you buy sweet or starchy snack foods in the winter and in the summer. This questionnaire will help you assess whether there is a seasonal rhythm to your weight gain and loss.

1. In which season(s) of the year do you tend to gain weight most easily? (Note: this does not refer to weight gain after holidays.)
fall   winter   spring   summer   no particular season

2. In which season(s) of the year do you tend to lose weight most easily?
fall   winter   spring   summer   no particular season

3. Do you eat more in the winter than in the summer?
yes   no

4. Do you crave more sweet and/or starchy foods in the winter than in the summer?
yes   no

5. Do you socialize less in the winter than in the summer?
yes   no

6. Do you find it harder to force yourself to exercise in the winter than in the summer?
yes   no

7. Do you find it harder to carry out your obligations in the winter than in the summer?
yes   no

8. Do you want to sleep longer in the winter than in the summer?
yes   no

9. Do you find it easier to eat a healthy diet in the summer than in the winter?
yes   no

10. Do you find yourself less tired in the summer than in the winter?

yes   no

11. Do you feel your mood becoming depressed or down or sad more often in the winter than in the summer?

yes   no

12. Do you find yourself acting more irritably in the winter than in the summer?

yes   no

If you answered yes to questions 1 and 2, then you have a seasonal pattern in weight gain and loss. To see whether these fluctuations are related to seasonal changes in mood, appetite, energy levels, and exercise, look at how many other questions you answered with a yes. If you also answered yes to questions 3, 4, 6, 9, and 10, then you should follow the two-part diet plan in Chapter Eight, diets for all seasons.

Some of you may gain weight in the winter but lose little of it in the warm months. The explanation for this could be as simple as not having the time, money, or interest to join a summer weight-loss program. If that is the case, you, too, should follow the seasonal weight-loss plan. Now you can use your summer months to lose weight, quickly and easily.

Some of you who suffer from winter weight-gain disorders may find yourself still gaining pounds *throughout* the rest of the year, not just in winter. Those of you who continue to gain weight during the summer could be affected by a number of other stresses, like having your children home for summer vacation, moving to another city, or entertaining too many relatives. Such pressures make it tough to lose weight at any time. In this case you should use the winter part of the food plan in Chapter Eight during the winter months to put the brake on weight gain. Then, instead of switching to the corresponding summer plan during the summer months, you should follow the serotonin-seeker's diet in Chapter Five. It will help you deal with summer stress and lose weight as well.

WHY ELSE ARE YOU GAINING WEIGHT?

Your responses to the following questions will point you to the appropriate chapter and food plan for your current overeating and stress needs.

Shift-Work Questionnaire

1. Are you currently working an evening or night shift?

   rarely   occasionally   often

2. Are you currently working an extended shift, so that your daytime job extends into the evening hours?

   rarely   occasionally   often

3. Are you working a second job or going to school at night?

   yes   no

4. Do you travel across time zones?

   rarely   occasionally   often

5. Does your job require you to wake up early or stay up late to deal with business in other time zones?

   rarely   occasionally   often

If you answered "occasionally" or "often" to any of the questions, read Chapter Nine on shift work. Although it has specific food plans and advice for those of you who work regular shifts, the information will assist anyone whose weight fluctuates in response to chaotic sleep and waking patterns. For example, if you travel across the United States to the Pacific Rim countries or to Europe and the Middle East occasionally or frequently for business, the suggestions on how to eat both to stay awake and to go to sleep will be helpful in controlling potential overeating.

Ex-Smoker's Questionnaire

The first two to four weeks after you stop smoking are the most difficult ones. That is the time when you are going to overeat; you will be experiencing the most severe cravings for nicotine and your mood shifts will feel intolerable. The smoking-withdrawal food plan is designed for this period; it will restore and reinforce serotonin levels so that cravings and mood can be controlled.

However, food cravings and the inability to control them may last much longer than a few weeks. If you use a nicotine patch, your cravings may shift as its dosage decreases. No one knows whether they will worsen with a smaller dose of nicotine or be the same as if you were not using the patch. This has not been studied.

You have to decide whether your cravings for sweet and starchy snacks are still being affected. One way is to ask yourself:

1. Do I feel the need to put food in my mouth every hour or so?

2. Do I ever wake in the middle of the night craving a cigarette?

3. Do I have a desire for sweet and starchy foods that is much greater than when I was smoking?

4. Is my mood still affected by lack of cigarettes?

5. Is my sleep still affected by lack of cigarettes?

6. Is my concentration and ability to work still affected by lack of cigarettes?

If you answer yes to any of these questions, try the smoking-withdrawal diet in Chapter Ten. Then, if you find that you don't need to snack as frequently or eat as much food as that diet calls for, switch to the serotonin-seeker's diet in Chapter Five.

After-Diet Binger's Questionnaire

The following questions will tell you whether your ability to control your eating is being lost along with weight as your diet proceeds.

1. Do you find it harder and harder not to cheat on your diet the longer you stay on it?

2. Do you fantasize about eating large quantities of foods you are not allowed to eat on your diet?

3. Are you becoming irritable, restless, impatient, tense, angry, and easily upset the longer you are on the diet?

4. Do you walk to the refrigerator fifteen times every evening after supper because you are not satisfied even though you are full?

5. Do you find excuses for not being able to follow the diet, such as travel, parties, social events, or business meals?

6. Have you stopped paying attention to portion sizes?

7. Do you feel too tired or grumpy to exercise?

If you answered yes to any of these questions, be sure to follow the eating instructions and food plan in Chapter Eleven, the after-diet eating plan.

SHOULD I EAT WHENEVER I FEEL STRESS?

By now you may be thinking that eating is the thing to do whenever you're not feeling happy. Of course that's not true; otherwise, every time you missed a green light or got caught in the rain or had a printer jam you would hightail it to the nearest doughnut shop counter or ice-cream store.

The food plans in this book are designed to maintain serotonin activity in the face of a large variety of stresses that can erode your serotonin stress-management system. If you follow the prescribed eating schedules, your biological need to "medicate" your stress by overeating will be eliminated. However, this does not mean that all your impulses to overeat will vanish. If, for most of your adult life, you have been unable to control your weight, there are probably other reasons you overeat—out of boredom, for example, or from social habit, like eating popcorn at the movies. You'll have to discover what is motivating you each time you are tempted to put something in your mouth when you are not hungry. The diet plans will increase your level of emotional comfort and make it easy to stop stress-driven eating, but you may also have to learn new eating behaviors in order to take advantage of your newfound calm.

Consider this example. Maybe you are doing some tedious desk work and want to take a break. In the past, you justified taking time off by telling yourself it was time for your snack. But you had a snack an hour ago; you really don't want to eat anything. What you want is a break. Habit takes you to the vending machine anyway. You need to understand that there are other justifiable reasons besides eating (stretching or relaxing, for instance) for putting your work aside for a few minutes.

Or maybe you are on an airplane. Hours before boarding you ate lunch from one of *The Serotonin Solution* food plans. You finished your snack just before boarding. However, when the flight attendant offers you another snack you eat it. Are you hungry? No. Are you eating because you're stressed? A second no—your snack took care of that. You're eating out of boredom, giving yourself something to do.

If you find yourself reverting to former overeating habits despite an improvement in your mood and the lack of any feeling of hunger, then you should seek the reason. If your problems seem overwhelming, should you find yourself in an extremely stressful situation such as divorce, for example, or if you are experiencing serious financial problems, or complex personal or work relationships, then you might consider seeking guidance. Help is available from numerous sources, including health professionals.

The serotonin-renewing remedies in this book will help you cope with your problems and help you avoid overeating in response to them, but the ultimate resolution may require some outside assistance. If necessary, the therapeutic effect of the diets can be amplified by counseling and support groups.

CHAPTER FIVE

The Serotonin-Seeker's Diet

The diet described in this chapter is the basic plan for anyone who cannot get through the day without nibbling or snacking in response to the stresses of daily life. It will ensure that the serotonin stress-management system is up and running all day long, but especially in the late afternoon and after dinner, those times of day when many of us are most vulnerable to stress-related overeating.

James is a typical serotonin seeker. He puts in long hours at his very demanding job as a professor at a Boston college, leaving for work early in the morning and rarely heading home until 6:30 P.M. But his evenings at home are hardly a time of quiet relaxation. In fact, at the end of each day, James simply shifts gears, trading the pressures of academia for the chaos of his large, bustling family of four school-age children. James's wife also works, and at the end of the day they share all the cooking, homework, and bedtime responsibilities. It's no wonder that the first place James heads after taking off his coat is the refrigerator. The serotonin-seeker's diet plan provides James with a stress-relieving snack on his way home from work and ends his nightly foraging.

Allison used to be too tired and stressed after work to even think about exercising. But after just a few weeks on the diet, she started working out regularly at her health club after work. Her late-afternoon carbohydrate snack lifted her mood and restored a sense of emotional well-being. Her peppier mood made it easier for her to decide to exercise rather than go home and become a couch potato.

The serotonin-seeker's diet plan contains a carbohydrate-rich snack and carbohydrate-rich dinner that are scientifically designed to promote maximal serotonin production and activity. It ensures that your serotonin stress-management system is working at full capacity at those times of the day when you are most likely to overeat because of stress. Think of the plan as "carbo-loading for stress."

You *must* eat the protein and carbohydrate components exactly as directed if you are to enjoy the benefits of our research. There is no flexibility here, so don't tamper with the recommended exchanges or servings. And don't be tempted to switch the timing of the meals, deciding that you'd rather eat the breakfast selections at dinner or trade dinner for lunch. If you do, you will not experience as much relief from your late-afternoon or evening stress. Not everyone experiences nighttime stress, however. For those of you whose stress-driven eating occurs only in the afternoons and who have no urge to overeat at night, I have provided a higher protein alternate to the dinner on the basic plan. But if the protein-rich conventional dinner leaves you psychologically hungry, switch to the carbohydrate comfort dinner.

A high-carbohydrate snack is an essential part of the diet. It will buffer you against stress and impulsive eating for about three hours, which should encompass the time of day when you feel most vulnerable to annoyance and frustration. The amount of carbohydrate prescribed for the snack is based on our MIT research. We now know how much carbohydrate must be eaten at one time in order to bring about a swift and effective surge of insulin, which, as you will recall from Chapter Two, is the substance responsible for rearranging the amino acids to the benefit of tryptophan. Although you will be tempted to skip the snack in the interest of saving a few calories, without it you cannot be sure that your brain will make enough serotonin. In other words, you run the risk of developing a carbohydrate craving and bingeing to satisfy it.

It is up to you to decide when to eat the snack. Choose the time of day when your eating control is most likely to be eroded by stress. This is a period when you typically experience psychological hunger and yearn for a sweet or starchy carbohydrate. If this happens several times a day, pick the moment when the feeling is at its most intense. Many people need to eat a carbohydrate late in the afternoon or right before dinner. This is an excellent time because your stomach will be relatively empty, the snack will be digested rapidly, and serotonin production will be boosted very quickly. If you want to add your snack to your carbohydrate comfort meal as a dessert, you can, but be aware of two things. If you eat a meal with more protein in it than recommended for the carbohydrate comfort meal and follow it immediately with the snack, the protein will prevent tryptophan from getting into the brain. Wait at least two hours after a high-protein dinner before eating your snack. A snack eaten early in the evening should exert its stress-relief effect until you go to bed if you normally are asleep by eleven or midnight. But if you are a night owl, your need for a soothing serotonin-boosting snack may last until one or two A.M. If this describes you, eat the carbohydrate comfort meal around seven or eight P.M.—and have the snack around ten P.M. Its effect should last until you are ready to sleep.

If you are one of those people whose need for a stress-relief snack arrives in the morning, by all means have it then. Keep in mind, however, that our experience at MIT showed us that nearly all our volunteers who claimed mid-morning psychological hunger were found to be experiencing actual physical hunger. These people ate very early breakfasts and late lunches, with too long a period in between. The solution for them was to eat lunch earlier, saving the snack for real symptoms of psychological hunger, which almost always arrived much later in the day.

The serotonin-seeker's diet provides approximately 1,400 calories a day or slightly less if you choose fat-free snacks. To some people, who are used to crash dieting, this may seem too many calories. To others, it may seem too few. It will, however, ensure two very important things: You will not feel deprived, and you will not feel crazed as you are losing weight.

Men in particular may find this calorie count too low, because of their larger muscle mass and greater energy expenditure. For them, the basic diet can be increased by as much as four hundred calories. The easiest and most healthful way to do this is to add additional servings of fruits or vegetables at the recommended times. (For instance, a large banana will contribute one hundred calories.) Men can also eat larger portions of the protein and carbohydrate selections, as long as they are careful not to alter the *ratio* of protein to carbohydrate.

Weight loss will occur fairly rapidly during the first week or two and then even out to about a pound a week after that. Because this eating plan is carbohydrate rich, your initial weight loss won't be as rapid as with some low-carbohydrate diets in which the rapid weight loss is really water loss. *On this diet the weight you lose will consist of fat, not water.* Besides, it is far better—not to mention more efficient in the long run—to lose weight slowly, feeling satisfied, than to always be longing for your next meal.

A special word to those who need to lose eighty pounds or more: If you find yourself hungry while on this diet, eat slightly larger servings. The difference between the number of calories you are used to consuming and those on the diet may be too great during the first two or three weeks. You may eat about three hundred additional calories a day from the vegetable and fruit exchanges without interfering with weight loss. If you are accustomed to more protein you may increase the serving sizes by one ounce, preferably at breakfast, the meal that contains the largest quantity of protein for the day. After your body becomes accustomed to taking in fewer calories, follow the portion sizes on the plan.

THE EXCHANGE LISTS AND HOW TO USE THEM

Unless you are a lifetime member of Weight Watchers and know exchanges better than your phone number, please read this section thoroughly and refer to it often. Even though many books, articles, and diet plans have been published using the food-exchange system, very few bother to explain what it is or how to use it. Once you understand it you'll find that it is quite easy to use.

Think of a food exchange as nothing more or less than a unit of measure, the same way an ounce, gram, or cup is a measure. What is being measured is nutritional content. All the foods that appear on a given exchange list have been grouped together according to their primary food value—that is, whether they consist predominantly of protein, fat, carbohydrates, or other nutrients (for example, vitamins). In a diet based on food exchanges, your food choices are determined not just by calorie counts but by nutritive values as well. If food choices were based solely on calories, a candy bar would have just about the value of a cup of cottage cheese. The difference between the two is only twenty or so calories. But the nutritional content of those foods, *per calorie eaten,* varies significantly.

The first food exchange is the protein group. This is called the meat/milk group in traditional exchange lists, since meat and dairy products are typical sources of protein and sometime in the dawn of weight-loss plan history, it was decided to name two exchanges after these foods. However, since the meat group contains dairy products such as cottage cheese and since a recent revision of exchange lists by the American Dietetic Association now puts milk into the starch group, I have decided that the exchange lists are more user-friendly if all high-protein foods are simply put into a protein exchange.

The starch/bread group contains foods that are high in carbohydrates. Breads, cereals and other grain products—rice, cornmeal, buckwheat, and wild rice—and starchy vegetables such as potatoes go into this group. There are also lists for fruits, vegetables, fats, and condiments (substances that enhance taste but have little caloric or nutritional value). The various exchange lists appear at the end of this book. Refer to the lists as you read through each of the other diet chapters. For your convenience I have also provided a carbohydrate snack exchange list, since it is crucial that you eat an appropriate sweet or starchy snack each day. This will help you choose snacks that are suitably high in carbohydrates and low in fat.

The exchange system offers you a way to design your own diet within the parameters of your chosen food plan. There are no "ideal" food choices here. As long as your meal and snack selections use the quantities and types of foods indicated on the exchange lists, you are staying on your diet.

For example, if you are allowed four carbohydrate exchanges in the carbohydrate comfort dinners, you can choose to get them from pasta, potatoes, bread, tortillas, or even pancakes. Your tastes determine what you eat; the food plan determines only the amounts of certain foods and when to have them.

For another example, the lunch guidelines specify three protein exchanges chosen from the protein group, two carbohydrates, and three vegetables, along with a selection from the free/condiment list. What this means is that you can choose to have a sandwich consisting of three ounces of turkey and two slices of bread spread with a small amount of fat-free mayonnaise, with lots of lettuce and tomato. Or you might prefer to have those same three ounces of turkey tossed with one cup of cooked pasta and an assortment of mushrooms and peppers. If you're on the run during lunch, you could opt for one cup of nonfat cottage cheese spread on rice cakes with a salad on the side or an assortment of crudités. If you can't face another slice of turkey, you can vary your menu to include two slices of nonfat ham and one slice of nonfat cheese stuffed into a baked potato and microwaved.

With just a little practice in the use of exchange lists, you'll find how very versatile your diet can be. If you like to cook, in a short time you will be able to combine selections from these exchange lists into delicious recipes. I've also taken some care to include some special selections for dining out on each plan's sample menus so you don't have to abandon your diet every time you go to a restaurant.

Food exchanges offer the easiest, most flexible way to adhere to a diet plan. With a little practice you'll find yourself becoming more familiar with the food groups and will know how specific foods fit into the plan. You'll find that using the exchange system is one of the most effective and satisfying ways of controlling your eating.

THE GENERIC EXCHANGE TABLE

The table below shows the different food groups and the nutritional components of each one. This is a generic list only, and the nutrient and calorie contents are averages. For a much more complete description of the foods in each category, refer to the exchange lists starting on page 266.

The Generic Exchange Table

ONE EXCHANGE   NUTRIENT AND CALORIE CONTENTS

Category	Carbohydrates	Protein	Fat	Calories
protein (1 ounce meat, poultry, or fish, or ¼ cup cottage cheese); milk (1 cup nonfat milk or 1 cup fat-free yogurt)		8 grams		70
starch/bread (½ cup of cereal, grain, or pasta)	15 grams			80
vegetables (½ cup cooked or 1 cup raw)	5 grams			25
fruit (½ cup juice or 1 cup raw)	15 grams			60
fat (1 teaspoon oil, butter, or margarine)			5 grams	45
condiments and "free" foods				based on food labels

Notice how foods have been grouped. The fat exchanges are easy to understand because their principal food value, that is, total percentage of their calories, comes from fat. The fruit exchange is also simple because fruit derives all its calories from carbohydrates. Starches like cereal, bread, and pasta derive their food value and calories from carbohydrates; and meat, poultry, fish, and dairy products like cottage cheese contain mostly protein. Choose lean meats and fat-free dairy products to reduce calories, and if possible eat yogurts that have had some of their sugar removed.

Food Labels

The labels that appeared on food packages a few years ago will make finding appropriate foods—especially snacks—simple. Check the gram counts on the labels against those specified in your chosen food plan. And you don't have to make yourself crazy: Just stay within two to five grams of the number called for in a particular exchange group.

Let's look, for example, at the labels for two different packaged foods and how they match up to the basic requirements of the snack exchange. Your daily carbohydrate snack is to consist of forty-five grams of carbohydrate, one gram or less of protein, and very little or no fat. The calorie content should be approximately 210. Following are food labels for two foods, pretzels and rice cakes, that show you how nutritional information is displayed on the new labels.

Gourmet Pretzels with Oat Bran (8-ounce bag) Nutrition Facts:

serving size:	1 ounce
servings per container:	8
calories:	104
calories from fat:	0
total fat: 0 grams	0 percent
saturated fat: 0 grams	0 percent

cholesterol: 0 milligrams   0 percent
sodium: 343 grams   5 percent
total carbohydrate 21.8 grams   8 percent
   dietary fiber: 3 grams   11 percent
   sugar: 4 grams
protein 1.37 grams

Butter-Flavored Rice Minicakes Nutrition Facts:

serving size: 7 cakes
calories: 60
total fat: 0 grams   0 percent
cholesterol: 0 grams   0 percent
sodium: 65 grams   3 percent
total carbohydrate: 13 grams   4 percent
protein: 1 gram

THE PROTEIN EXCHANGE

The portion sizes on page 73 refer to foods that are cooked or canned. Because cooking removes water and fat, cooked food will weigh less. If you aren't sure about how much a particular food will shrink, weigh it after cooking.

Some foods, like peanut butter and hard cheeses, which contain substantial amounts of fat along with protein, are not included on this list. Instead, they can be found in the fat exchange. And although eggs are a good source of high-quality protein, they should not be eaten as a protein exchange more than once or twice a week (unless your physician has told you not to worry about your cholesterol intake). On the other hand, many high-fat protein foods, formerly forbidden on diets, now exist in low-fat and low-calorie versions. These include hot dogs, sausages, and luncheon meats made from poultry rather than pork or ham; ricotta (an essential ingredient of lasagna), which is now available in a fat-free form; and many hard cheeses that are also now made with less fat. New lower-fat versions of many other foods are constantly entering the supermarket; look for them.

Dairy products are an excellent source of protein as well as calcium. To stretch your calories and control your fat intake, select low-fat or fat-free dairy foods. If you don't like either milk or yogurt by themselves, you can use them and other dairy products as ingredients in various recipes. For example, use low-fat or fat-free ricotta in pasta dishes, add nonfat milk to pudding mixes, or prepare milk-based clam and corn chowders. Buttermilk (made from nonfat milk) can be mixed with pureed vegetables in soups, and yogurt is a good substitute for sour cream on potatoes or in salad dressing.

However, give yogurt a chance on its own. Fat-free sugar-reduced yogurts now come in a seemingly inexhaustible variety of flavors. You'll be amazed at how good so few calories can taste.

Some of you avoid dairy products because you have trouble digesting lactose, or milk sugar. Millions of people lose the ability to digest lactose when they reach adulthood, and suffer from gastrointestinal distress when they drink milk or eat cheese or ice cream. In recent years, lactose-free or 70 percent lactose-free milk products, including cottage cheese, have become available. There are also pills, which you swallow prior to eating, that contain the enzyme that digests lactose. And, of course, there are milk substitutes, such as soymilk.

Protein

1 exchange equals:
1 ounce (cooked) lean meat, poultry, or fish
$^1/_2$ cup nonfat cottage cheese
1 ounce lowfat cheese
8 ounces (1 cup) skim milk
8 ounces (1 cup) nonfat yogurt

THE STARCH EXCHANGE

Today there seems to be a nearly endless selection of starchy foods available, from oatmeal to tortillas. No list of these foods can be comprehensive, so check labels to see how a food not on the list in this book will fit into the exchange system. If a starchy food is prepared with fat, it obviously will contain more calories than its nonfat counterpart. French fries or hash brown potatoes cooked in oil have more calories than baked potatoes. When choosing your starch exchanges, opt for the low-fat or nonfat versions.

Recently, many starchy and sweet foods have been reformulated to remove or decrease their fat content. It is important to note that just because fat has been removed doesn't necessarily mean the food is low in calories. Gigantic fat-free muffins can have as many calories as their fat-containing smaller-sized cousins. So check the calorie content of fat-reduced starchy and sweet foods. Also check the portion size. Based on the promotional copy on the label, you might think a particular food is extremely low in both fat and calories—until you see what one "serving" consists of. If the label on a "diet" muffin tells you that a "serving" is only one hundred calories but the muffin itself consists of six servings, that's *not* a low-calorie muffin.

Starch

1 exchange equals:
4 ounces ($^1/_2$ cup) cooked cereal, grain, or pasta
1 ounce (1 thin slice) bread
$3^1/_2$ ounces ($^1/_3$ cup) cooked beans, peas, or lentils

THE VEGETABLE EXCHANGE

Although all vegetables are good for you, not all are created equal in terms of nutrients. They differ considerably in their vitamin and mineral contents. One carrot, for example, can satisfy your vitamin A need (in the form of beta-carotene) for a day. An entire head of iceberg lettuce provides only minor amounts of vitamins and minerals. Green and orange vegetables pack the biggest nutritional punch, with purple (beets and eggplant) and red (tomatoes) following. Dark green leafy vegetables, such as spinach or kale, are rich in folic acid; winter squash is high in beta-carotene. Pale-colored vegetables (like cucumbers and zucchini and other summer squashes, mushrooms, iceberg lettuce) tend to be full of water and not too much else.

While it is commonly assumed that fresh vegetables contain more nutrients than frozen and canned ones, you should consider where you live in relation to where the vegetables are harvested. For instance, if you live at the tip of New England and the vegetables are coming from the bottom of Chile there probably isn't that much difference between the nutrients in a "fresh" carrot and one that is "fast frozen." Do not plan on eating unlimited quantities of vegetables just because they are good for you. Calories add up, so stick to the portion sizes as given in the exchange list as much as you can. With the exception of water-dense vegetables such as cucumbers, lettuce, radishes, summer squash, and sprouts, unlimited servings of vegetables may increase your calorie intake above the allowable limit.

Vegetable

1 exchange equals:
$1/2$ cup cooked vegetables
1 cup raw vegetables

THE FRUIT EXCHANGE

Fruits, like vegetables, supply us with a variety of vitamins and minerals. For instance, citrus fruits are rich in vitamin C; apricots and bananas contain potassium. Many fruits and vegetables are high in fiber, a food constituent that is in short supply for those who eat a diet heavy in processed food. Fiber keeps the process of digestion working. Follow the guidelines for the number of fruit servings carefully; their calorie contents are generally higher than those of vegetables and can add up quickly. Avoid fruits canned in sugar syrup. An important point to remember is that fruit does not make a satisfactory stress-relief snack. Even though its fructose (fruit sugar) is a carbohydrate, it does not have any impact on the transport of tryptophan to the brain. An apple a day may do a lot of good things for you, but it can't keep the stress at bay.

Fruit

1 exchange equals:
1 small- to medium-sized piece of fruit
$1/2$ cup unsweetened fresh fruit juice
$1/2$ cup unsweetened canned fruit juice
$1/4$ cup dried fruit

THE FAT EXCHANGE

Everyone needs to eat a certain amount of fat each day. However, since so many foods naturally contain some fat—meats, cheeses, breads, eggs, and so forth—you don't have to add much extra fat to your diet. On the other hand, fat is a flavor enhancer, and when used sparingly can make a mediocre dish outstanding. Use fat the way you should use salt and you will not overeat it. When selecting a fat, try to pick one that is relatively healthful, such as olive oil or other unsaturated fats. With the exception of palm oil, a common ingredient in many packaged foods, oils are healthier sources of fat than solid, or saturated, fats like butter, shortening, or margarine. That is because liquid fats are monosaturates (like olive oil) or polyunsaturates (like canola, peanut, or walnut oil) and are associated with a smaller increase in LDL (popularly called "bad") cholesterol in the blood.

Fish oil, or the fat found naturally in fish such as salmon or mackerel, is especially good because it contains the beneficial omega-3 fatty acid. Recently, walnuts were found to be beneficial to the cardiovascular system, so go ahead and add them in small amounts to crunch up a salad or perk up some fat-free cottage cheese.

Do cut down on your fat intake whenever possible by using fat-free substitutes for foods such as mayonnaise, salad dressings, cream cheese, sour cream, and margarine. Be wary of "reduced fat" foods. Some are still very high in fat, so read the package labels carefully.

Fat

1 exchange equals:
1 teaspoon butter, margarine, or oil

THE CONDIMENTS AND "FREE" FOODS EXCHANGE

Condiments are foods that contain less than twenty calories per specified portion and yet can make the difference between a "blah" meal and something great. Some, like tarragon, thyme, and cinnamon, you can eat in unlimited quantities because their calorie content per serving is negligible. Others, like garlic, chives, scallions, shallots, and ginger, have a higher calorie content. But since the recipes limit the amount you can add of these, you won't have to count calories.

"Free" foods are those that look and smell like the real thing but don't necessarily taste like it—and *aren't*. Some of these "fake" manufactured foods taste quite good. Your local supermarket will have salad dressings, mayonnaise, sour cream, cream cheese, and margarine in low-fat or no-fat versions that are much better tasting than similar products available just a few years ago. The proliferation of such foods will allow you to eat those formerly "forbidden" foods.

However, in making selections from the "free food" list, be sensitive to the fact that these foods do contain *calories*—even if they don't contain any fat. Check labels carefully. If a single "serving" has less than twenty calories and that's all you are eating—for example, a tablespoon of salad dressing—help yourself. But if you are eating more than twenty calories' worth, you must check the exchange lists to see where the product belongs and how many exchanges it amounts to. For example, if you are eating baked potato chips—the low-fat version of traditional potato chips, which are fried—you can count them as your carbohydrate snack. But be sure to check the starch list to see what amount will add up to the forty-five grams of starch allowed for the snack.

THE BEVERAGE EXCHANGE

Although water is not on the exchange list, it should be drunk in adequate amounts: eight 6- to 8-ounce glasses a day, or the equivalent in other noncalorie-containing liquids. Alcohol, soda, juice, and milk all have calories. Carbonated water, or seltzer, does not; it is just water charged with carbon dioxide.

Here are the exchange guidelines for each meal on the basic serotonin-seeker's diet, with suggested menus that can be followed at home and in many restaurants.

Note: If you cook dishes with multiple ingredients, use a cookbook that gives you counts for calories, protein, carbohydrates, and fat for each recipe. More and more cookbooks, and recipes that appear in newspapers and magazines, now provide this information. Do this even if you are an experienced cook until you become familiar with what you are actually eating.

BREAKFAST

All your life you have heard that breakfast is important. It's true. As the name tells you, it is the meal that breaks the fast your body has been on for an average of ten to twelve hours. If you eat wisely, breakfast will nudge your body into mental and physical action, accelerate your metabolism to daytime (as opposed to sleeping) levels, and supply a substantial amount of needed daily nutrients. In the serotonin-seeker's diet, breakfast has a special role: It is the meal where you are least likely to overeat due to stress. This is not to say that you will never feel stressed upon awakening. If you have children, the demands made upon you during the first hour after awakening can make the job of an air traffic controller seem like a stroll in the park. Nevertheless, most people somehow manage to get through those first few hours without giving way to impulsive overeating. Maybe it is due to the fact that the body is primed to handle more during the early part of the day, so it can deal with the problems that come its way with a minimal erosion of its stress-relief system.

Thus, breakfast on the plan is not a stress-relief meal. It is designed with one purpose only: to nourish. The meal may contain more protein than you are accustomed to eating, especially if your breakfast usually consists of a muffin or bagel and a cup of coffee. If you find it difficult—or even distasteful—to eat the amount of protein recommended on the breakfast exchange list first thing in the morning, you can make a change. Split the meal into two smaller ones. The first can be eaten when you get up, and the rest sometime later in the morning.

Breakfast Exchanges

2 protein (16 to 18 grams)
1 starch (15 grams)
1 fruit (15 grams)
total calories: 280

Sample Breakfasts

yogurt-fruit sundae (1 cup fat-free sugar-free yogurt mixed
with ¹/₂ cup fat-free ricotta, 3 tablespoons Grape-Nuts
sprinkled on top, with ³/₄ cup fresh berries or ¹/₂ banana,
sliced)
Equals: 2 protein, 1 starch, 1 fruit

or

farmer's breakfast:
1 egg cooked any style (if fried or scrambled use nonstick spray)
1 turkey sausage
¹/₂ English muffin
1 teaspoon jelly
Equals: 2 protein, 1 starch, 1 fruit

or

yogurt shake (2 cups fat-free banana cream pie yogurt
blended with 1 banana, sliced)
Equals: 2 protein, 2 fruit

or

morning melt (2 slices fat-free cheese, 1 ounce low-fat turkey
"ham," and one 3-ounce pita, heated until cheese
melts)
¹/₂ cup orange or grapefruit juice
Equals: 2 protein, 1 starch, 1 fruit

or

breakfast crunch (1 cup fat-free ricotta, 1 small apple, sliced
on top of ricotta, sprinkled with 1 teaspoon cinnamon,
1 teaspoon sugar, and ¹/₂ cup low-fat granola)
Equals: 2 protein, 1 starch, 1 fruit

or

two-part breakfast:
Part 1: 1 cup fat-free cereal, 1 cup milk: eat at home
Part 2: 1 container fat-free sugar-free yogurt, 1 peach or
    orange: eat at work
Equals: 2 protein, 1 fruit, 1 starch

Note: If you like to sleep late on weekends and holidays, you can combine breakfast and lunch calories and exchanges into one brunch. Eat the meal late in the morning.

LUNCH

Try to adhere to the lunch food choices as closely as possible. You may be eating this meal away from home. Therefore, planning what, where, and when you eat is very important. Whatever your food choices, keep the following tips and general principles in mind.

Speed up planning and preparation time by eating the same foods every day. While this might seem like a rather punitive suggestion, keep in mind that most of us do it naturally, dating back to our school days. Remember eating peanut butter and jelly sandwiches week after week? I know a woman who successfully lost a lot of weight (as an adult, of course) by going to a very pricey restaurant and ordering the same meal day after day. It worked for her because her decision about what to have was made; all she had to do was eat it. Lunch staples such as canned tuna, microwaveable soups, turkey and chicken cold cuts, mock crabmeat, nonfat cheese, frozen vegetable mixtures (which can be thawed and mixed into the starchy component of your meal) are all easy-to-find, inexpensive foods that can make regular appearances on your lunch menu.

Buy peeled, cut-up vegetables. If you have access to a salad bar or a restaurant that sells salads or an assortment of raw or cooked vegetables, get your selection there. Bring your protein from home (see above) and add it.

Microwaveable soups, stews, meals, and leftovers are always possible lunch options. There is also a large variety of dehydrated low-fat or nonfat soups containing carbohydrates such as lentils, beans, and potato-vegetable mixtures. Add some cut-up slices of lean beef or chicken and you have a perfectly respectable meal.

If your schedule does not assure you of an appropriate place to have lunch every day, plan ahead, or else you'll find yourself running into fast-food restaurants and ruining your best intentions. Carry a thermos of hot soup along with some cans of tuna or chicken in your briefcase or car.

When eating out, make your needs known: Insist that mayonnaise, butter, salad dressing, and cream be kept to a minimum or be eliminated altogether. Before ordering, inquire about portion sizes. If servings are large, choose an appetizer that contains protein, share a main course, or eat only half and take the rest home. (For example, an average main course in a fish restaurant is six ounces—twice as much as allowed on the lunch protein exchange.)

Lunch Exchanges

3 protein (24 grams)
2 starch (30 grams)
2 vegetable (10 grams)
1 condiment and "free" food
total calories: 420

Restaurant Options

Fast-food restaurant: grilled chicken sandwich with salad. If you wish, you can substitute a baked potato for the roll.

Coffeeshop or diner: baked potato plus salad and grilled chicken fillet (no roll).

Bagel shop: any flavor bagel with smoked or regular turkey breast; *or* bagel with low-fat tofu spread plus one cup beef vegetable or chicken noodle soup, or minestrone soup and small Greek salad. If the bagels are so large that they require two hands to hold they may weigh as much as four ounces—or almost twice as much as the bagel on the exchange list. Eat just half; otherwise you will be going over both the starch and calorie limits.

Mexican restaurant: burrito with chicken, sautéed peppers and onions, beans (only if not cooked in lard); *or* shrimp burrito in salsa verde; *or* black bean salad (again, no lard) composed of beans, onions, peppers on a bed of greens

American restaurant: salad Niçoise, a fancy tuna and vegetable plate (use vinegar or fat-free salad dressing, and skip the bread if potatoes are included in this dish); *or* seafood salad; *or* sliced turkey or lean roast beef sandwich; *or* Oriental chicken salad; *or* steamed vegetables (baked potato on the side); *or* chicken salad in pita bread (check out the dressing). If French fries come with any of these meals, request pita, whole wheat bread, rice, or a baked potato instead.

Japanese restaurant: barbecued salmon or chicken marinated in teriyaki sauce with rice; *or* noodles with shrimp, chicken, or fish; *or* casserole of salmon and assorted vegetables in broth (ask for rice); *or* steamed chicken with mixed vegetables and rice; *or* mixed steamed vegetables with tofu and rice

Packaged Microwaveable Meals

Stouffer's three-bean chili melt with one slice fat-free cheese plus raw vegetables and a glass of skim milk; *or* Stouffer's cheese ravioli plus raw vegetables and one cup fat-free sugar-free yogurt; *or* Stouffer's angel-hair pasta plus two ounces of cooked chicken or turkey and one piece of fruit; *or* Stouffer's Oriental beef with vegetables and rice plus one cup fat-free sugar-free yogurt and $1/2$ cup strawberries; *or* Knorr potato leek soup plus three ounces cooked chicken or turkey or smoked turkey luncheon meat and vegetables or fruit.

CONVENTIONAL DINNER

If you follow this plan, make sure you know the portion sizes of what you are eating. Because this plan is so similar to the way you probably eat now, you may not bother to check the size of your portions. Also, by getting used to seeing what four ounces of cooked beef or one half cup of fruit looks like, for instance, you will be able to judge serving sizes in restaurants and on buffet tables.

The Conventional Dinner Exchange

3 protein (24 grams)
1 starch (15 grams)
2 vegetable (10 grams)
1 fruit (15 grams)
2 fat (10 grams)
total calories: 490

Here are some recipe suggestions for carbohydrate comfort dinners.

CARBOHYDRATE COMFORT DINNER

Dinner on the serotonin-seeker's diet is designed to satisfy your psychological as well as physical hunger. High in carbohydrates, it should effectively boost serotonin levels for at least three hours, especially since it will be preceded or followed by a carbohydrate snack. The combination of this snack and dinner is the most effective means of relieving stress, renewing your eating control, and satisfying both types of hunger. Because the portion sizes of the protein and starch components of this dinner are the reverse of what you normally eat at dinnertime, weigh and measure food during the first five or six days of the diet. Otherwise, you may find yourself eating too much protein and too little carbohydrate.

If you are cooking for others who are not following this diet, you will find it easier to prepare a conventional meal. This consists of a main course protein like chicken, a starch like rice or potatoes, and vegetables and fruit. Serve yourself large amounts of the starchy food and very small amounts of the protein.

If you are eating in a restaurant or find yourself in a social situation where you cannot control what is being served, do the same thing. Nibble at the protein and make sure you have enough starch. If no starchy side dish is served, then eat bread or rolls to satisfy the starch exchange requirement. In a restaurant, don't be shy about asking for extra bread or ordering a plain baked potato or pasta without butter, olive oil, or cream. Of course, when you are a guest in someone's home it can be trickier. If you don't want to draw attention to your eating, then tell your hostess ahead of time that you are following a low-protein diet.

If you are eating alone, you can dine on pancakes, waffles, French toast, hot cereal, vegetarian chili, or pasta, and forget about the chicken breast in the back of the refrigerator.

However, finding microwaveable dinners that will work on the dinner plan is not so easy. Most of these prepared meals contain too much protein. There are pasta or rice dinners that, when combined with your own protein and vegetables, make a fine dish. For instance, I recently rediscovered frozen blintzes (thin crepes wrapped around various fillings), which, to my surprise, are a lot lower in calories than I thought. Two potato blintzes can make an interesting change from the usual starch. Gnocchi, an Italian potato-based dumpling, is another example of a frozen food that, served with tomato or mushroom sauce, can become the basis of a different, delicious meal. Check out new items in your supermarket's freezer, many of which will come from foreign cuisines. Some (like the blintzes and gnocchi) are high in carbohydrates and low in protein.

If you use a lot of microwaveable or frozen meals, check serving sizes carefully. Often the picture on the package shows a deceptively ample-looking serving. If you find that the actual meal is very small, providing you with less food than you need, supplement the packaged dinner with enough food to meet your starch, vegetable, and protein exchanges.

Because so many diets are based on exchanges, many packaged dinners provide exchange information on their labels. Look for it.

Dinner Exchanges

1 protein (8 grams)
3 starch (45 grams)
2 vegetable (10 grams)
1 fruit (15 grams)
2 fat (10 grams)
total calories: 510

Sample Carbohydrate Comfort Dinner Menus

two 6-inch pancakes or two slices of French toast
1 tablespoon lite pancake syrup
$1/2$ cup nonfat cottage cheese
1 cup chopped melon
Equals: 1 protein, 3 starch, 1 fruit, 1 fat

or

4 potato blintzes (cooked with nonstick spray)
1 cup fat-free yogurt mixed with chopped chives, $1/2$ sweet
    red pepper, $1/2$ cucumber, and 2 to 3 radishes
1 cup unsweetened applesauce
Equals: 1 protein, 3 starch, 1 vegetable, 1 fruit

or

$1^1/_2$ cups cooked pasta
1 ounce turkey or chicken (left over or part of family dinner)
    or 1 turkey sausage
$1^1/_2$ cups packaged stir-fry vegetable mixture
2 teaspoons olive oil
2 tablespoons Parmesan cheese
oregano and pepper to taste
Equals: 1 protein, 3 starch, 2 vegetable, 2 fat

or

1 large baked potato stuffed with 1 ounce turkey or chicken
(leftover or part of family dinner) and $1/2$ cup salsa,
warmed
1 cup strawberries
1 cup steamed spinach tossed with 1 teaspoon olive oil
2 cinnamon WASA crackers
Equals: 1 protein, 3 starch, 1 fruit, 1 fat

RECIPES

Spaghetti Carbonara

This is an example of how a basic pasta can be dressed up with selections from the free list to add satisfying flavor without adding
fat and calories.

Serves 1

$1^{1}/_{2}$ cups uncooked spaghetti
1 serving egg substitute
2 tablespoons grated onion
1 clove garlic, crushed
1 teaspoon imitation bacon bits
2 teaspoons grated Parmesan cheese
coarsely ground black pepper

Cook the spaghetti according to package directions. Meanwhile, combine the egg substitute, onion, garlic, and bacon bits.
When the pasta is done, drain, but do not rinse. Add the egg
mixture to the pasta and toss lightly, until the strands are
coated. (The heat from the pasta will "cook" the egg.) To serve,
sprinkle with Parmesan cheese and lots of coarsely ground
black pepper.

Pasta with Mushrooms and Prosciutto

The Italian ham prosciutto combines meat and fat exchanges to give your comfort dinner an authentic taste of Italy. If prosciutto is not readily available in your area, substitute 2 slices Canadian bacon or boiled ham.

Serves 1

    1¹/₂ cups pasta, uncooked
    ¹/₂ cup fresh mushrooms, any variety
    2 thin slices prosciutto, cut into strips
    ¹/₂ cup diced onion
    vegetable cooking spray

Cook the pasta according to package directions. Meanwhile, spray a nonstick skillet with vegetable cooking spray. Over high heat, sauté the remaining ingredients until the mushrooms are tender. Toss together with pasta and serve.

Note: Some varieties of fresh mushrooms give off more juice than others. If the mixture seems dry, add a tablespoon or two of water to the skillet.

Pasta with Tuna, Fresh Basil, and Olives

A grown-ups' tuna casserole that can't be beat when fresh basil's in season. Olives are high in oil, so count them as at least one fat exchange. If adding more than four olives, adjust your later fat consumption accordingly.

Serves 1

    1¹/₂ cups cooked pasta
    1 ounce of tuna packed in water, drained
    1 clove garlic, crushed
    ¹/₂ cup fresh basil leaves, shredded

2 sundried tomatoes, drained and sliced into thin strips
4 Greek-type olives, pitted and diced

Toss ingredients together and serve warm or cold.

Couscous with Lamb and Vegetables

Lamb has a wonderful flavor that can add richness to a dish without adding fat. This exotic offering will make you forget you're dieting. For an even more authentic flavor, add your dinner fruit exchange to the main course and sauté 1 small diced apple along with the vegetables.

Serves 1

1 ounce ground lamb
1 small zucchini, cut into chunks
4 scallions, including tops, sliced
1 medium tomato, diced
1 to 2 tablespoons cooking sherry (or water)
1½ cups couscous, prepared according to package
    directions
1 tablespoon curry powder, or more, to taste

Sauté the lamb and vegetables together in a small skillet until lightly browned, adding 1 to 2 tablespoons of water or cooking sherry as necessary to prevent sticking. Add couscous and curry powder and mix well.

Lunchtime Nachos

A great choice for those who bring their lunch to work or have access to a microwave.

Serves 1

25 nonfat tortilla chips
2 slices nonfat cheese or 2 ounces fat-free cheese spread
$^{1}/_{2}$ cup salsa
2 ounces canned beans or $^{1}/_{4}$ cup bean dip

Arrange tortilla chips on a microwave-safe plate; top with cheese, salsa, and beans.
Microwave on high for 2 minutes.

Dinner Stuffed Potato 1

A well-stuffed potato is more than the latest in fast-food fads; with a little imagination and a microwave, it can be a dieter's dream.

Serves 1

1 large baked potato
1 ounce turkey or chicken, shredded
$^{1}/_{2}$ cup salsa
1 tablespoon fat-free sour cream

Slit potato lengthwise and mash the insides lightly. Top with chicken or turkey, salsa, and sour cream. Microwave on high for 90 seconds.

Dinner Stuffed Potato 2

Serves 1

1 large baked potato
$^{1}/_{4}$ cup nonfat cottage cheese
1 scallion, including green top
2 tablespoons plain nonfat yogurt
1 tablespoon fresh herbs, such as basil, parsley, sage, chives

$^1/_2$ teaspoon powdered garlic
1 teaspoon imitation bacon bits

Slit the potato lengthwise and mash the insides lightly. In a food processor or blender, whirl together remaining ingredients. Stuff the potato and microwave on high for 60 to 90 seconds.

THE SNACK

You must follow three guidelines faithfully.

1. Eat one carbohydrate snack daily, either before dinner or at mid-evening.

2. The snack must contain a minimum of forty to forty-five grams of carbohydrates and a maximum of 210 calories. Fat-free snacks are your best bet, because they have a low calorie count. Eating this much carbohydrate in such a limited number of calories is easy these days because of the large number of fat-free carbohydrate snack foods available. According to food industry reports, the fat-free snack food market is the fastest growing segment of the food industry. Expect to see many more fat-free products in the next few years.

3. The snack cannot be fruit. It has to be a sweet or starchy carbohydrate that will stimulate insulin, but it can be *anything* that falls within the carbohydrate and calorie guidelines. Do not feel guilty about your choice. You are eating the snack for its effect on your mood and mental energy levels, not its nutritional value. So enjoy. While the list below is far from being complete, it will point you in the direction of the types of snacks you can eat. Check package labels for portion sizes and refer to the snack section of the starch exchange lists (page 270) for more options. Remember: Let your taste buds *and* the carbohydrate and calorie contents be your guide.

Snack Options

- Breakfast cereals. The sugar-sweetened fat-free kind taste wonderful if you are looking for a crunchy, sweet taste. Do check the amount you are allowed before you start dipping your hand into the box, otherwise you will almost assuredly eat more than you need.
- Fat-free tortilla chips. There are new brands available all the time.
- Rice cakes. These have come a long way since they first appeared. If you gave up on them years ago, give them another taste. Some are excellent.
- Crunchy snacks. Try baked potato chips, baked potato crisps, rice puffs, fat-free pretzels and animal crackers, bagel chips, and pita chips.
- Fat-free pastries. Nearly every cookie and cake that was traditionally made with fat is now available in a fat-free form.
- Sweets. There are many chewy candies that are fat-free, including saltwater taffy, licorice, candy corn and pumpkins, gumdrops, jelly beans, all types of gummy candies, and nougats. Do not, however, rely on hard candy, lollipops, or dietetic candy for snacks. Hard candies must be sucked slowly and take too long to take effect. Dietetic candy will leave you unsatisfied because it doesn't contain sugar.

Chocolate will not satisfy your cravings unless you have it in a low-fat or fat-free form like Tootsie Rolls, chocolate-flavored licorice, or chocolate jelly beans. Chocolate contains a substantial amount of fat in the form of cocoa butter. And, although it is this fat that gives chocolate its meltingly lovely feeling in the mouth, the fat content means chocolate takes longer to digest. So, even though your taste buds will thank you, your serotonin-seeking brain cells will be waiting a very long time. And you run the risk of continuing to eat while you are waiting for your psychological hunger to be satisfied.

AVOIDING TROUBLE

Even with the best of intentions, you serotonin seekers may run into trouble if you don't keep these troubleshooting tips in mind:

- Be prepared. What works for the Boy Scouts will also help your dieting efforts. Anticipate what and where you will be eating during the day and plan for it. Take charge of meal and snack planning to avoid situations in which you have nothing—or nothing appropriate—to eat.
- Respect portion size. The fastest way to jeopardize weight loss is to ignore the amount of food you eat.
- Slow down; you're probably eating too fast. Select foods that need to be chewed—baked potato skins, coleslaw, beans, spaghetti, shredded wheat, Grape-Nuts, and lean meat.
- Sip, don't gulp, a beverage while you are eating.
- Experiment with spicy, low-fat condiments as substitutes for high-fat spreads and sauces. Salsa, peppery or garlicky jelly, Chinese dipping sauces, honey-flavored mustard, and marinated or pickled vegetables will tantalize your taste buds without adding many calories.
- A little wine, if consumed in moderation, can enhance the calming effect of dinner, as well as prolong the time you take to eat it. One ounce contains about one hundred calories. Wine spritzers (wine mixed with seltzer) are a good choice.
- Take a daily vitamin and mineral supplement as insurance against those days when you're not able to eat high-quality vegetables and fruits or the variety of whole grain products you should be eating.
- Never substitute an artificially sweetened beverage for your snack. When the body craves carbohydrates it wants sugar, not an artificial sweetener.
- Before you go to a dinner or cocktail party, eat some of the food allowed on the exchange list for that meal. Make sure you have your snack, too, if the time you would normally eat

it coincides with the event. Your appetite will be blunted, making it easier for you to refrain from filling up on fattening appetizers or eating the large portions of food that invariably are presented. Be sure to remember what you ate before leaving home. Mentally subtract it from what you are being served so you don't overeat.

- Be sure to exercise. Physical activity of any type helps to work off stress by easing muscle tension and soothing angry feelings. To be most effective, exercise should be vigorous; you should feel your heart beating more quickly and your breathing become more rapid. A slow stroll won't do much to dispel irritation, anger, or frustration, but a fast trot, slow jog, or quick ride on an exercise bicycle for even five minutes, will dispel your bad mood and promote calmness. If you can, follow your exercise with a hot or whirlpool bath, or a steam bath or a sauna. You will feel even better.

  Exercise uses up calories, which translates into quicker weight loss. In addition, you increase muscle, or lean body, mass. The more muscle you have, the more calories you burn up, even when resting. This is probably why men, who have proportionately more muscle than women, can lose weight so much more quickly.

  Whether you exercise or not and how much you do is, of course, a matter of self-discipline and motivation, state of muscle and bone fitness, health, and time. Exercising regularly takes commitment. But, for those who begin and stick with it, there will be extraordinary benefits.

There will be times when you will find the diet plan hard to follow. You may not want to pay attention to portion sizes, you might be tired and bored with planning meals and snacks, and you might very well resent having to adhere to a schedule and avoid tempting fattening foods. If any of these happen there are two things to do:

1. Go back and review Chapter Four. See if you are experiencing any of the additional stress triggers described. If so, turn to the chapter or chapters that describe your particular triggers—

PMS, winter depression, or whatever—and follow the relevant diet plans.

2. Read Chapter Thirteen on how to control binge damage. This will remove guilt as one of your overeating triggers and allow you to get back on to the diet plan.

CHAPTER SIX

The
Stressed-Mommy Diet

Ask any stay-at-home mother of a young child and she will likely tell you the same thing: Motherhood brings enormous joy as well as bottomless exhaustion and unrelenting stress. It also brings weight gain. Preparing, serving, and cleaning up after an endless round of meals, with few outside activities to distract you from the comforts of the refrigerator, causes the inevitable: Your toddler is now toilet trained but you still cannot get back into your prepregnancy clothes.

One obvious cause is the lack of a support system. If you do not have a live-in nanny, cook, housekeeper, and/or therapist, you must cope with the unending crises alone. Your baby has just fallen asleep after three hours of screaming and then his sister has a tantrum. Your two-year-old thinks the bathtub is her potty, and your four-year-old thinks her sibling should leave home—permanently. You have spent thirty minutes cutting up vegetables so your three-year-old will start eating something other than Cheerios, and he pretends to gag on the carrot slice you entice him to try.

Even grandmothers are not immune. A patient of mine took

care of her working daughter's two preschool children for a week after their baby-sitter quit without warning. One child was going into the "terrible twos," and the other was emerging (but not very quickly) from the equally troublesome fours. One wanted to eat all the time, while the other was extremely picky and fussed. On top of this the weather was cold and rainy, which meant they were housebound, and the grandmother felt completely isolated because she didn't know anyone in the neighborhood. The result: seven pounds gained in one week.

Unless you have incredible self-discipline, it's all too easy to succumb to the pernicious combination of stress, exhaustion, and ready access to the refrigerator, and eat too often—and too much. If you are a stressed-out mommy, the following behaviors will be all too familiar to you:

1. spending most of your waking hours in the kitchen
2. nibbling whenever you have some free time
3. eating the leftovers your children leave on their plates
4. eating to keep yourself going emotionally
5. eating when you wake up at night because of the children
6. eating more when you must stay indoors
7. sitting on a playground bench, watching your children and eating their snacks because you are so bored
8. eating because you are angry at your husband for not helping out enough around the house
9. dipping into the cookie jar when your children's constant whining, bickering, and temper tantrums become too much
10. eating to keep yourself awake when you are extremely tired
11. eating to give yourself an excuse for relaxing

WHY CAN'T I LOSE WEIGHT?

If all that picking and nibbling has made you put on weight, you have probably tried to diet, thereby adding to your stress. You've learned that conventional diets just won't work for you: They not only take away calories but also remove the foods that comfort you and help you cope. Their primary appeal is being able to get out of the house to go to a weekly diet meeting.

I believe that the stay-at-home mommy is susceptible to chronic emotional stress. Look at it this way: If your body is constantly exposed to viruses and bacteria and you are barely over one viral or bacterial illness before you are exposed to another, you may be constantly sick because your immune system cannot cope. In the same way, if you are continually bombarded by all the details of nonstop child care, your brain serotonin may not have a chance to recover from dealing with one stress before being faced with the next one and the one after that and so on. And, as we now know, when the brain needs to make more serotonin, the body demands that you eat carbohydrate-rich foods.

Mothers of young children are particularly in need of edible tranquilizers. They need foods that decrease their susceptibility to stress, increase their tranquillity and patience, and allow them to enjoy and cope successfully with the demands of child rearing.

It is possible to lose weight and satisfy the brain's demands for serotonin, even in the face of constant stress. My customized weight-loss plan will allow you, the stressed mommy, to wear your prepregnancy wardrobe again, as well as help you regain your emotional equilibrium.

The main principle of the diet is simple: Eat mainly carbohydrates before the sun goes down, and eat protein at night.

The plan provides between 1,400 and 1,600 calories a day, depending on the number of snacks you eat. There will be days when it will be impossible for you not to snack continuously because of excessive demands on your coping powers. On such days, extra food may be crucial, so figure on the higher calorie count and follow the suggestions under Extra-Hard Days (see page 112). While you might not lose weight on those days, you won't gain any either.

THE STRESSED-MOMMY DIET

Breakfast

Be sure to eat your own. Resist the temptation to eat your child's leftovers for this or any other meal. If early mornings are chaotic, wait until the kitchen traffic subsides and the children are playing, napping, or willing to leave you alone for fifteen minutes. Then sit down and eat. Otherwise you will find yourself eating much more than you should.

Breakfast Exchanges

1 protein (8 grams)
2 starch (30 grams)
1 fruit (15 grams)
optional: coffee or tea
total calories: 290

Sample Breakfast Menus

1 cup fat-free breakfast cereal
1 cup nonfat milk
$1/2$ cup orange juice
Equals: 2 starch, 1 protein, 1 fruit

or

1 English muffin
1 cup fat-free sugar-free yogurt
$1/2$ banana, sliced
Equals: 2 starch, 1 protein, 1 fruit

or

1 low-fat toaster tart
$1/4$ cup nonfat pineapple cottage cheese

1 tangerine
Equals: 2 starch, 1 protein, 1 fruit

or

1 fat-free fruit-filled breakfast bar
1 cup nonfat milk
$1/2$ banana, sliced
Equals: 2 starch, 1 protein, 1 fruit

or

2 thin slices toast
$1/4$ cup plain nonfat yogurt spread
2 teaspoons sugar-free jelly
Equals: 2 starch, 1 protein, 1 "free" food

Lunch

Do not skip this meal. You will have been working all morning; your body needs to be nourished. Take the time to enjoy your food and sit down to eat. You don't allow your children to eat standing up; neither should you.

Lunch Exchanges

1 protein (8 grams)
2 starch (30 grams)
1 vegetable (5 grams)
total calories: 255

Sample Lunches

tuna roll-up ($1/4$ cup water-packed tuna mixed with 1 table-
    spoon fat-free mayonnaise and 1 chopped tomato, $1/2$
    chopped scallion, 1 chopped carrot, packed into 6-inch pita)
Equals: 1 protein, 2 starch, 1 vegetable, 1 "free"

or

1 turkey hot dog
1 hot dog bun
1 carrot, sliced
1 cucumber, sliced
pickle slices
Equals: 1 protein, 2 starch, 1 vegetable

or

1 baked potato stuffed with 2 slices fat-free cheese and 1 red
    pepper, sliced, microwaved
Equals: 1 protein, 2 starch, 1 vegetable

or

1 cup microwaveable vegetable-noodle soup (containing 110
    to 180 calories) with 1 ounce cooked chicken, beef, or
    low-fat luncheon meat added
1 tomato and cucumber, sliced
Equals: 1 protein, 2 starch, 1 vegetable

or

1 small toasted bagel
1 slice low-fat luncheon meat
1 slice fat-free cheese
mustard
tomato, lettuce, cucumber, and pickle garnish
Equals: 1 protein, 2 starch, 1 vegetable

Mid-Afternoon Snack

Choose a snack that contains about forty grams of carbohydrates and no more than two hundred calories. Be sure to select
very low-fat choices. Have a cup of tea, coffee, or cocoa (in-

clude the calories and carbohydrates in cocoa in your snack allowance), put your feet up, and relax. Do this even if you have only ten minutes. This snack time is essential for promoting peace of mind and peace in the house. The serotonin-boosting effect of the snack will make coping with your children's late afternoon acting out much easier.

Early Dinner with Children

This mini-meal should be eaten if you feed your children and put them to bed before you have dinner with your partner. If the children have their dinner with the grown-ups, then skip this meal and add the exchanges to those on the adult dinner plan (page 104). However, both you and your children may need to eat something early in the evening if you normally dine fairly late. By 7 P.M. you will have been working for twelve hours or more and will likely need to eat again. And if the interval between the children's afternoon snack and dinner is more than a couple of hours, they will be so tired by the time dinnertime rolls around that they won't eat. An early mini-meal around 5 or 5:30 P.M. will ensure that some dinner will be eaten by your children and will prevent you from nibbling continuously until your dinner is on the table.

Early Dinner Exchanges

1 protein (8 grams)
1 starch (15 grams)
1 vegetable (5 grams)
total calories: 175

Sample Menus for Early Dinner with Children

1 carrot, sliced, cooked with 1 teaspoon brown sugar and a
     pinch of nutmeg
1 small boiled potato sprinkled with parsley and 1 teaspoon
     olive oil

1 cup cocoa made with nonfat milk
Equals: 1 protein, 1 starch, 1 vegetable, 1 fat

or

1 slice Boboli pizza (with the equivalent of 2 slices fat-free
cheese and reduced-fat tomato sauce with no more than
1 teaspoon olive oil)
salad with fat-free salad dressing
Equals: 1 protein, 1 starch, 1 vegetable

or

1 cup vegetable soup
2 cheese-flavored fat-free rice cakes
1 serving fat-free sugar-free pudding made with nonfat
milk
Equals: 1 protein, 1 starch, 1 vegetable

or

1 hard-boiled egg mixed with chopped green pepper,
scallions, fat-free mayonnaise, and mustard
1 slice whole wheat toast
Equals: 1 protein, 1 carbohydrate, 1 vegetable

Adult Dinner

If it is at all possible to eat a quiet, adults-only dinner at least two
or three nights a week, do so. It will give you the chance to eat a
complete meal uninterrupted. Dinner provides most of your
daily protein needs because I expect (and hope) that by this time
the children are asleep. Your serotonin-based stress-management
system will no longer be tasked. If, however, you have a teething
or otherwise distressed child, choose a menu from the will-this-
day-never-end section instead. Those menus contain carbohydrate meals and should sustain and, if necessary, increase

serotonin levels to help you remain tranquil—even if your child is not.

Adult Dinner Exchanges

3 protein (24 grams)
1 starch (15 grams)
3 vegetable (15 grams)
2 fat (10 grams)
total calories: 455

Sample Menus

1$\frac{1}{2}$ cups stir-fry vegetables with 3 oz. skinless chicken breast and $\frac{1}{2}$ cup rice
Equals: 3 protein, 1 starch, 3 vegetable

or

beef stew with winter vegetables and dumplings:
3 ounces lean beef
1$\frac{1}{2}$ cups mixture of carrots, winter squash, and parsnip
2 small dumplings
Equals: 3 protein, 1 starch, 3 vegetable

or

1$\frac{1}{2}$ cups spaghetti squash with tomato sauce and 3 ounces turkey meatballs
$\frac{1}{2}$ slice garlic bread, made with fat-free margarine and garlic powder
Equals: 3 protein, 1 starch, 3 vegetable

or

3 ounces baked cod with topping of bread crumbs, lemon, and 1 teaspoon olive oil

1$^1/_2$ cups steamed spinach
1 small ear of corn
Equals: 3 protein, 1 starch, 3 vegetable, 1 fat

or

1 low-fat taco shell filled with 3 oz. ground turkey cooked with
onion, jalapeño pepper (to taste), and green pepper topped
with shredded lettuce and 1 slice grated fat-free cheese
Equals: 3 protein, 1 starch, 3 vegetable

Will-This-Day-Never-End? Dinner

Since this meal will be eaten when you have the time, the menu
selections are based on quick and simple preparations. Some of
the foods have an added virtue: They can be eaten while you are
pacing with a baby on your shoulder or sitting with a child on
your lap.

Will-This-Day-Never-End? Exchanges

1 protein (8 grams)
4 starch (60 grams)
1 fruit (15 grams)
2 fat (10 grams)
total calories: 540

Sample Menus for Will-This-Day-Never-End? Dinner

2 teaspoons peanut butter
$^1/_2$ banana, sliced
1 large raisin bagel
1 container fat-free pudding
Equals: 1 protein, 4 starch, 1 fruit, 2 fat

or

2 slices fat-free cheese on 6" pita, melted in microwave
1 cup unsweetened applesauce
Equals: 1 protein, 4 starch, 1 fruit

or

2 cups instant oatmeal with $1/4$ cup mixture of raisins and
    dried apricots
1 cup apricot-flavored fat-free sugar-free yogurt
Equals: 1 protein, 4 starch, 1 fruit

or

4 toaster waffles spread with $1/2$ cup apple butter or 1 cup
    applesauce
1 container of fat-free sugar-free vanilla yogurt
Equals: 1 protein, 4 starch, 1 fruit

or

1 cup blueberries
2 cups sweet breakfast cereal
1 cup fat-free sugar-free vanilla blueberry yogurt; shake it
    and drink (add a little nonfat milk to make shaking
    easier)
Equals: 1 protein, 4 starch, 1 fruit

or

1 container microwaveable noodle soup
4 cheddar cheese-flavored rice cakes
1 banana
$1/2$ cup pineapple-flavored cottage cheese
Equals: 1 protein, 4 starch, 1 fruit

Here are some recipe suggestions for stressed-mommy dishes.

RECIPES

Summer Camp Favorite Beans

This kid favorite can be a diet pleaser, too. Note how low-fat Vienna sausages made with chicken substitute for the traditional high-fat franks. Most canned baked beans now come in low-fat and vegetarian versions, so be sure to check the nutrition label.

$1/2$ 13-ounce can low-fat or vegetarian baked beans
2 Vienna-type sausages, made with chicken, cut up
1 tablespoon ketchup or barbecue sauce
2 teaspoons yellow mustard
$1/2$ packet NutraSweet type sweetener
dash hot sauce

Combine ingredients over low heat and serve.

Baby Food Soups

Those jars of baby food your little darling refuses can help you toward a slimmer, more serene you.

Broccoli Cheese Soup

Serves 1—Eat as 1st course

1 6-ounce jar Gerber's Broccoli, Carrots and Cheese
    Dinner
8 ounces low-sodium chicken broth
$1/2$ teaspoon dried thyme
Salt and pepper to taste

Combine the above ingredients in a small saucepan, heat, and serve.

Butternut Squash Soup

Serves 1—Eat as 1st course

> 2 4-ounce jars strained butternut squash
> 4 ounces low-sodium chicken broth
> 4 ounces evaporated skim milk
> 1 chopped apple
> Garlic and onion powder to taste
> Salt and pepper

Combine the above ingredients in small saucepan, heat, and serve.

Fruited Yogurt Soup

Serves 1—Eat as 1st course

> 2 4-ounce jars strained fruit such as peaches, pears, or bananas
> 1 6-ounce carton plain yogurt
> Fresh mint for garnish

Combine fruit and yogurt and chill. Garnish with mint as desired.

Mom's Stir-Fry Special

A late-night dinner in a dish.

Serves 1

> 3 ounces lean beef, cut into thin strips
> 2 cloves garlic, minced
> 1¹/₂ inch slice fresh ginger, grated
> 1 medium onion, sliced thin
> 2 generous tablespoons soy sauce
> 1 tablespoon red wine vinegar

1 teaspoon peanut butter
1 10-ounce package Oriental stir-fry vegetables
$1/2$ cup cooked rice

Marinate the pork, garlic, ginger, and onion in the soy sauce and vinegar for at least one hour in the refrigerator. Spray a skillet or wok with nonstick vegetable spray and heat over medium heat until it sizzles when a drop or two of water is added. Melt the peanut butter in the skillet. Remove the marinated mixture from the refrigerator and add it all at once, including any liquid, to the pan. Stir fry for three to five minutes, or until the meat loses any pink color. Add the vegetables, stirring to blend, and continue cooking until slightly tender but still crisp. Add the rice and cook just until heated through. Serve with additional soy sauce, if desired.

AVOIDING TROUBLE

1. Do not skip meals. Eat them even if they are delayed. If you don't, you will be less able to resist stress-induced impulsive overeating—bingeing, in short.

2. Sit down and enjoy your food.

3. Eat high-fiber foods such as whole grain breads, pastas, bran-type cereal, and fibrous vegetables like carrots and broccoli.

4. Never skip a snack in order to save calories. You will more than make up for it by eating too many calories later. If you are overeating snacks, then you may be waiting too long to eat them. Have the snack sooner rather than later in order to build up serotonin levels and make you less vulnerable to stress.

5. Take a vitamin-mineral supplement daily. If you eat few or no dairy products, take a calcium supplement or three or four calcium-based antacid tablets. You need about eight hundred milligrams of calcium daily.

6. Drink at least six cups of water or other noncaloric beverages daily.

7. If you still feel like eating at the end of a meal, pop a rich-tasting hard candy in your mouth or suck on a lollipop. Either will keep you from nibbling on the leftovers as you clean up.

8. Remove temptations: Keep junk foods out of the house and don't use your children as a justification for having them. If anything, the children should be a justification for *not* having them, since you don't want your children to form bad eating habits.

9. Never eat your kids' leftovers.

10. Make time to relax and eat your snack. If your children seem glued to you, try this: Keep a box of special toys, books, games, or videos that they can use only while you are having your private time. Take these special items away again when you emerge feeling calmer. After a few days your children will be asking you to go away and rest so they can play with their treat.

EXERCISE

Yes, I know you've heard the word *exercise* before, but look at it this way: You are already exercising several body parts when you carry groceries, your children, and their strollers. Your arm muscles are probably much stronger now than they were before you had children. The same thing is true of your leg muscles. You probably walk miles every day even though it may be just around the house or the supermarket.

The best way to accelerate weight loss and decrease your stress is to exercise aerobically. This means moving fast enough to break a sweat and increase your heart rate. And the best way to look good is to tone those sagging body areas.

Ideally, the best way to accomplish both is to go to a health club or gym that provides machines like treadmills, stair step equipment, exercise bicycles, rowing machines, and aerobic classes and a pool. Or you can jog, roller-skate, or bicycle several times a week. Increased muscle mass will not only make you look slimmer but also will help you slim down faster. Calories burned doing aerobic activities will speed up weight loss.

Realistically, however, most of you will find many of the above suggestions difficult to follow because of the necessity of juggling baby-sitters, schedules, and, of course, unanticipated crises.

There is an effective fallback position: home exercise. Think about all the exercise you already do and build on it. Walk more; don't drive if your destination is less than three-quarters of a mile away. Put the kids in the stroller and/or backpack and walk. If they are old enough they can walk, too. Use your bike when weather permits and fasten a child seat onto it.

If you used to run, consider getting a stroller you can push while you jog. And run—do not walk—after your toddler. If you can afford to do so, buy or rent an exercise bicycle, stair stepper, or treadmill. Too expensive? Buy an exercise video and follow it.

Do you have an old jump rope handy? Five minutes of skipping will speed up your heart rate, make you warm and sweaty, and work off those calories. Engage your children's interest by teaching them jump rope jingles or have them count your jumps. (I had a neighbor who became so proficient at jumping rope that all the neighborhood children used to gather in her backyard to watch her.)

If your children are old enough, they can help you with toning and stretching exercises. Have one hold your legs while you are doing sit-ups. Have another count repetitions.

Finally, don't forget seasonal activities such as raking leaves, washing windows, shoveling snow, gardening, filling bird feeders, weeding, cleaning out the garage, and maintaining the outside of your house. All of it counts as exercise.

EATING RIGHT ISN'T THE ONLY THING THAT MATTERS

Vulnerability to stress and the overeating it produces can be minimized if you schedule some relief time. If you miss daytime adult conversation, see if your community has any activities that put you into contact with other mothers. Use your phone: Get a long extension cord or a cordless phone so you can talk while doing chores or trailing your toddler as he or she races through the house. Hearing another adult voice can turn a lonely afternoon into a tolerable one. Make recreational or social time for yourself by going out for an evening or afternoon. If you have to be relentless about getting a sitter, then do: Ask friends, relatives, and local teens. Look into baby-sitting services at the local Y, health club, church, synagogue, or community center. Sign up for local play groups, library reading sessions, backyard camps during summer vacations, and supervised playground activities. Preschool music, art, and nature programs also exist. Seek them out.

Your diet is very important for its role in replenishing and nourishing your serotonin-management system. However, it is imperative not to overlook emotional, intellectual, and social nourishment as well. All will work to get you back in shape and feeling much better faster.

EXTRA-HARD DAYS

Some days the serotonin boost you will be getting from the regular diet plan just won't be enough to control your eating and decrease your stress. There is, however, a way to prevent a sleepless night or multiple crises before 7:45 A.M. from inciting you to eat half a cake for breakfast—and the rest before lunch.

But first you must recognize your eating is out of control. If you deny you are eating impulsively or try to excuse it without dealing with it, the day will be lost.

Instead, admit you do not want to stick to your diet that day (I promise you, lightning will not strike) and then follow this how-many-hours-left-until-the-kids-go-to-bed? plan.

1. Have foods available for all-day nibbling.
2. Make sure the foods are of the kind to maximize serotonin levels.

Begin by gathering all the foods you know you'll want to nibble; that is, the foods you know you would be able to avoid if this were a more normal day and you could stick to your diet. Put all these items on your kitchen table. Individual tastes vary, but it's likely your choices will include some of the following: peanut butter, ice cream, cookies, potato chips, frozen cookie dough, muffins, popcorn, cereal, jams, crackers, chocolate chips.

Next, remove all the really fattening foods. For example, if you have both frozen yogurt and ice cream on the table, return the ice cream to the freezer. Eliminate butter-rich cookies, crackers, or oily snacks like potato chips. These foods will really sabotage your diet; and if you've successfully avoided them recently, you may not be able to digest them easily and will end up feeling nauseated or bloated.

Take some small zip-top sandwich bags and fill them with the foods you've decided you can eat. For instance, put chocolate-covered raisins in one bag and sugared breakfast cereal in another. Fill one bag with miniature marshmallows, another with pretzel sticks, and a third with fat-free chocolate cookies. Foods like frozen yogurt, marshmallow topping, fat-free fudge sauce, or other spoonable goodies can be stored in the freezer or refrigerator in individual juice glasses or empty baby food jars. Make yourself two sandwiches of peanut butter (go easy on this) and jam or honey, cut them in eighths, and place them in sandwich bags. If possible, crumble, break, or cut other food items into tiny pieces before putting them in the bags. Break large pretzels into small pieces; take a rolling pin or the edge of a large knife and smash the cookies into small pieces; use scissors to cut pita bread into tiny wedges. That way, once you begin to nibble, the smaller the size of what you eat, the fewer calories you will ingest. Popcorn is another good nibbling food, as are any fat-free or very-low-fat potato, tortilla, flavored-rice, or vegetable chips. Certain breakfast cereals, like Rice Krispies and Grape-Nuts, are perfect for this type of eating.

After you've cut, crumbled, and otherwise prepared and packaged all your choices for the day, put all the foods that you haven't refrigerated in one big basket and place it where your children can't get at it. This is your supply of food until you go to sleep. You cannot add to it, but you do not have to eat it all either. Once you've seen everything you're allowed to eat, you may decide that eating all of it isn't that important.

Every time the urge to eat hits, reach into the basket and take out a sandwich bag or remove a filled juice glass from the refrigerator. If you leave the house, take some sandwich bags with you. Do not eat anything that you have not already packaged.

After a while, your hand will tire of putting cookie fragment after cookie fragment into your mouth, and you will find yourself losing interest in eating any more. Don't, however, try to stuff a handful into your mouth all at once just because you've gotten tired of eating one piece at a time. These foods will just spill out of your hand and onto your clothes and the floor.

Obviously, you are not going to lose weight on such a day. More important, however, is that you are planning and exerting control over your eating. Even though you may be eating much more than you should, you are *not* eating impulsively. You know exactly what you are eating. You have created a selection of foods tailored to your tastes and designed to calm you and increase your coping power.

Tomorrow, as they say, is another day. You will probably want to return to your regular eating program then. And you will go back to it with confidence, because *you* have asserted your power.

CHAPTER SEVEN

The Mind-Over-Menstrual-Cycle Diet

Premenstrual syndrome (PMS) has many faces. According to the gynecologists who do research on the causes of and therapies for PMS, it may produce as many as two hundred different symptoms, ranging from breast tenderness, bloating, and cramping to restless sleep, irritability, memory and concentration lapses, anger, confusion, fatigue, increased or decreased energy, and, as we know, uncontrollable, intense food cravings, especially for sweet or starchy foods. Four percent of the women with PMS undergo severe changes in mood, appetite, and a sense of physical well-being, sometimes becoming unable to carry out their usual work, family, and social obligations. Millions of others suffer lesser but still draining, demoralizing, and occasionally debilitating changes. Symptoms may persist for up to fourteen days or even longer, beginning around the time of ovulation and letting up only one or two days after the onset of a period. Or they may be short-term, beginning only three or four hours before a period starts. Some women even get a preview of their symptoms on the day they ovulate, experiencing mood and appetite changes that last for a few hours but do not actually settle into a premenstrual pattern for several more days.

Surveys estimate that about twenty-five million women suffer every month from PMS. Even that number may be an underestimate, because these figures seem to be based only on the women who complained of symptoms to their doctors and whose doctors believe, on the basis of what may sometimes be overstrict diagnostic criteria, that their patients really do have PMS.

As prevalent as this syndrome is, and despite decades of research, no one yet knows why it occurs in some women and not in others or why symptoms vary so greatly. According to a recent issue of the *New England Journal of Medicine*, the extreme variability in PMS susceptibility cannot be accounted for by hormones, because PMS occurs in women with normal hormonal function. Comparisons of hormonal patterns reveal no apparent differences in hormone function between women who experience PMS and those who don't.

One of the few things we do know is that PMS seems to be experienced more often as women enter their thirties. Many women report they started to have PMS after having children. However, it is not clear whether pregnancy itself has an effect on PMS, or if pregnancy simply happens to coincide with the time in a woman's life when PMS symptoms are most likely to manifest or to increase in severity.

RESEARCH ON PMS

Research on PMS has followed two paths. One is focused on finding ways to help women who suffer from physical symptoms such as nausea, headaches, painful preperiod cramps, intense sleep disturbances, muscle aches, and other ailments. Unfortunately, the remedies that work best to alleviate these symptoms are also the most radical: They involve drugs that induce a type of chemical menopause.

The other research path has focused on mood disruption—premenstrual depression, agitation, and anxiety. For some women these symptoms can be as debilitating as the physical manifestations are for others. It is now assumed that separate and distinct systems in the body are responsible for the physical and emotional symptoms of PMS. Unfortunately, the remedies used to relieve one have little effect on the other.

A breakthrough in treating the depression and agitation of PMS was reported in the spring of 1995. Prozac, along with other antidepressants that increase the availability of serotonin in the brain, relieved the most severe mood changes of about 60 percent of the women treated. There is, however, a major issue still to be resolved. In order for the drugs to be effective during the latter part of the cycle when PMS symptoms appear, they may have to be taken throughout the cycle. Current research is now focusing on whether or not antidepressants can be taken only as needed and still have the same effect; in which case the prescription would probably be for medication to begin right after ovulation, or mid-cycle, and continue until menstruation begins. Since these are powerful drugs, the less a woman has to take of them, the better, especially since the women who take them are of childbearing age. Women who become pregnant while on one of these drugs may unknowingly expose their fetuses to risks that are still not documented or understood. For this and other reasons the benefits of drug therapy for women who do not suffer from severe premenstrual mood changes may not outweigh its possible risks.

PMS AND FOOD CRAVINGS

For many women, there is one common indicator of PMS: an increased appetite for sweet or starchy carbohydrates. And although this change in eating habits is only one in the range of unpleasant premenstrual events, it carries, literally, a great weight. Because of it, these women will not be able to control their eating and will probably gain weight.

Despite the frequency with which this problem occurs, it has received little attention from either research laboratories or weight-loss programs. In fact, I know of only one commercial weight-loss program that recognizes the need to alleviate premenstrual stress. Unfortunately, the "therapy" this program offers is a vitamin supplement that has been shown in many scientific studies to be worthless.

I myself have long been extremely interested in the problem of premenstrual stress and overeating—both personally and professionally. Like many women, I have had insatiable food cravings and have felt debilitated enough by PMS to have had to rearrange my schedule to avoid burdening myself when I knew coping would be a chore. So all the women who come to me for weight-loss counseling, as well as the female volunteers in our studies, are asked whether they experience PMS. If they do, we ask if their symptoms include mood changes and impulsive overeating. At least half these women claim their moods and eating patterns change drastically before they get their periods.

As one particularly articulate woman put it: "I feel like Dr. Jekyll and Ms. Hyde. During the first half of my cycle I have no trouble following the diet and, in fact, no trouble exercising every day. I never feel hungry; I never have any unsatisfied cravings. But about five or six days after I ovulate I feel as if my body is possessed by another entity, one who can't stop eating. I start shoveling food in as soon as I wake up. All day long I have one thing on my mind: When can I eat more chocolate, more ice cream, more cookies. And forget the exercise. If I manage to walk to the corner store to replenish my stash of chocolate chips I consider myself doing very well."

THE BEST REMEDY FOR PMS: FOOD

Paradoxically, the best treatment for the increased appetite and impulsive overeating of PMS is food. The urge to eat during the days preceding menstruation is brain driven. While it is not yet understood how this happens, the monthly shift in hormones affects several neurotransmitters, including serotonin. As a result, the serotonin stress-management system functions abnormally, causing the emotional distress and impulsive overeating that plague so many women.

Food seems to be nature's remedy for these natural monthly changes in emotional state and appetite. The challenge for both a dieter and a woman trying to maintain her weight is to choose the right foods for the job and eat them at the right time and in the appropriate amounts. Unfortunately, when premenstrual carbohydrate cravings occur, the usual impulse is to instantly grab something sweet or starchy, which will very often be loaded with fat. But as you read in Chapter Three, fatty foods take longer to digest than carbohydrates, and any serotonin-regulated relief of emotional distress will be a long time coming. And you will continue to eat many brownies, candy bars, and slices of pizza while waiting for the carbohydrates to be digested and sent into your bloodstream.

Until recently, no information was given to women on how to use sweet or starchy foods to subdue carbohydrate cravings and relieve emotional distress. Instead, women were advised to avoid carbohydrates, especially the sweet ones. But that advice was wrong. The premenstrual diet plan I have developed makes effective use of high-carbohydrate low-fat foods to reverse the changes in serotonin function caused by premenstrual shifts in hormones, and thereby restore control over impulsive overeating.

THE RESEARCH BEHIND THE REMEDY

Several years ago I collaborated with Dr. Amnon Brzezinski, a gynecologist from Israel, on a series of studies that examined how food choices change during the menstrual cycle among women who suffer from PMS. We wanted to observe the role that serotonin played in causing dramatic swings in appetite.

Women who suffered from premenstrual syndrome lived in our Clinical Research Center for three days at the beginning of their cycles when they were symptom free. They came back for three days at the end of their menstrual cycles, when PMS-induced changes in mood and appetite were at their height. We also studied women who had never experienced PMS to see whether their eating habits differed from those of the women with PMS.

All the volunteers ate their meals from the same selection of protein and carbohydrate foods described in Chapter Two (see page 25), and all snacked from the computer-linked vending machine that was also described in Chapter Two. At the beginning of their menstrual cycles, the women ate moderate amounts of food at meals and snacked very little. When they were premenstrual, however, they not only ate considerably more starchy foods at meals, they nearly wore a groove in the floor, padding their way to and from the vending machine. Though the machine was stocked with a variety of protein and carbohydrate foods, the snacks they chose consisted invariably of sweet or starchy snack foods. When we analyzed the results, we found the volunteers with PMS increased their intake by about five hundred calories a day, with almost all those calories coming from sweet and starchy carbohydrates.

Why were the women who had PMS eating so many carbohydrates when they were premenstrual but not earlier in the month?

The answer was found, once again, in serotonin. In one study in which our volunteers were treated with dexfenfluramine or a placebo for three months, the drug had a dramatic effect on their mood and overeating. They felt better and stopped overeating. Consuming a high-carbohydrate dinner of cornflakes and sugar had a similar effect. Ninety minutes after they ate the cereal, the volunteers all felt an improvement in mood.

The best nondrug option for battling PMS cravings is food, in the kinds and amounts prescribed by the special diet I've developed.

THE MIND-OVER-MENSTRUAL-CYCLE DIET

This food plan is designed to keep the serotonin stress-management system operational even in the face of PMS-induced disruptions.

It should be used only on days when you experience premenstrual food cravings, along with high levels of irritability, anger, agitation, confusion, spaciness, or depression. Since it provides about three hundred to four hundred more calories than the serotonin-seeker's diet (depending on whether you have the optional evening snack), it is a weight-maintenance, not weight-loss, program, with the emphasis on preventing overeating.

In order to make sure that you anticipate and recognize the symptoms of PMS before they drive your eating out of control, you need to know when you will be entering the premenstrual phase of your cycle. So track your cycle each month. The first day of your period is considered day one. Ovulation usually occurs anywhere from day eleven to day fifteen. For most women their period begins about twelve to seventeen days after that. This means the premenstrual time of the month can begin anywhere from day fifteen to day twenty-seven or twenty-eight. Complicating the situation even more is that the length of a woman's cycles can vary from month to month.

But if one day you begin to fantasize about one-pound chocolate bars, bags of spicy potato chips, and hot fudge sundaes, and you become so grumpy and irritable that even your dog crawls under the bed to get away from you, these are excellent indicators of PMS. Check your calendar. If you see that your period is expected anytime within a one-day to two-week period, then that's your signal to switch to this diet.

Of course, every woman has her own internal tracking system and usually can tell from month to month when she is premenstrual. But sometimes the mood and appetite changes can occur so suddenly that she is not prepared for them and may not recognize them, which is why keeping a record can be helpful.

Take the example of June, a college professor. She told me of the time she attended a university gala dinner, virtuously sitting through one barely eaten course after another—with only one thing on her mind: chocolate ice cream. She was so obsessed that dinner table conversation, speeches—all went unheard. As soon as dessert (untouched strawberries and cream) was over she made a dash to the nearest ice cream store, where she inhaled a double dip chocolate brownie ice cream cone.

"This *never* happened to me before," she told me. "I actually thought I was losing my mind. I've heard of people having hallucinations—but for chocolate! That night I was looking over my calendar and noticed that my period was due the next day. 'So *that's* what this is all about,' I thought. If I had only checked my calendar sooner I would have eaten the chocolate ice cream before going to the dinner and been able to act like a responsible faculty member, instead of a chocolate-crazed zombie."

You may not experience the premenstrual cravings and mood changes with the same intensity day after day prior to your period. For some women the appetite and mood changes are mild at first and then intensify, reaching a peak right before the period begins. For others, there are good days interspersed with premenstrual days. And still others will have good/bad/good days, making sort of a checkerboard of symptoms during the latter part of their cycles.

USING THE MIND-OVER-MENSTRUAL-CYCLE DIET

You can start the diet any time you feel you need it. If you become aware of premenstrual changes in the late morning or afternoon, begin the diet at lunch or dinner. Don't wait until the next day.

The therapeutic doses of carbohydrate snacks are spaced at short enough intervals to make sure their effects don't wear off before the next snack is eaten. And the type of foods recommended for meals will enhance the comforting and appetite-controlling effects.

Another important reminder: Don't weigh yourself during your premenstrual time. Since you are apt to retain water then, the weight shown on the scale will tell you how much water you are retaining, not whether or not you are losing fat. From long experience most women can expect at least a two- to five-pound loss of weight after their periods start.

SAMPLE PMS MEAL AND SNACK MENUS

Breakfast Exchanges

2 protein (14 grams)
2 starch (30 grams)
total calories: 300

Breakfast

2 scrambled eggs (or low-fat egg substitute)
1 slice of fat-free cheese
2 slices raisin toast
1 teaspoon jam
Equals: 2¹/₂ protein, 2 starch, 1 "free"

or

microwave melt (1 small pita or mountain bread, 2 slices
    ham-flavored turkey luncheon meat, 2 slices fat-free
    cheese)
Equals: 2 protein, 2 starch

or

1 cup of fat-free pineapple cottage cheese
¹/₂ cup fat-free granola
¹/₂ banana, sliced
Equals: 2 protein, 1 starch, 1 fruit

Lunch Exchanges

1 protein (8 grams)
3 starch (45 grams)
1 vegetable (15 grams)
total calories: 335

Lunch

1 slice swiss cheese
1 large slice pita bread (6 inch)
1 carrot
$^1/_2$ tomato
pickles
1 red pepper, diced
1 tablespoon fat-free mayonnaise
1 cup fat-free potato chips
1 glass fat-free chocolate milk
Equals: 1 protein, 4 starch, 1 vegetable, 1 "free," 1 fat

or

1 large baked potato
$^1/_2$ cup fat-free plain yogurt mixed with scallions and cucumbers
1 glass fat-free chocolate milk
2 fat-free cookies
Equals: 1$^1/_2$ protein, 3 starch

or

1 bagel, sliced
$^1/_4$ cup yogurt spread*
1 tablespoon honey
1 glass fat-free chocolate milk
Equals: 1 protein, 3 starch, 1 "free"

Mid-Afternoon Snack

45 grams carbohydrate
1 fruit
total calories: 280

*recipe on page 155

5 caramel-coated or apple cinnamon fat-free rice cakes
1 glass apple juice

or

2 fat-free cupcakes
$^1\!/_2$ cup strawberries

or

1 fat-free muffin
1 orange

Dinner Exchanges

1 protein (8 grams)
3 starch (45 grams)
2 vegetable (10 grams)
1 fruit (15 grams)
1 fat (5 grams)
total calories: 465

Dinner

1 bowl of canned corn or potato chowder made with low-fat
   milk
1 cup oyster crackers
1 orange
1 cup of mixed green salad
Equals: 1 protein, 3 starch, 1 fruit, 2 vegetable

or

1 cup stir-fried vegetables
2 cups Chinese noodles
1 ounce cooked chicken

1 tangerine
Equals: 1 protein, 3 starch, 2 vegetable, 1 fruit

Evening Snack

30 grams carbohydrate
total calories: 120

chocolate marshmallow sandwich (2 graham crackers, fat-free
    chocolate syrup, and 3 marshmallows) microwaved
    briefly

or

1 cup fat-free chocolate ice cream
1 tablespoon of marshmallow topping

Follow the food exchange guidelines and the suggestions below to make sure that you are getting the nutrients you need.

If you are not interested in eating full servings of fruits and vegetables when you are premenstrual, you should try to incorporate them as ingredients in your main course. Including vegetables is easy. Add some frozen vegetables to your beef noodle soup while it's cooking; make a pizza with low-fat cheese and broccoli; bake a potato and top it with steamed vegetables and fat-free yogurt; fill a pita with small amounts of tuna, chicken, or mock seafood salad and add vegetables; or top noodles or spaghetti with stir-fried vegetables or mix them into a bowl of rice.

Vegetables, such as corn, kidney beans, chickpeas, potatoes, and green peas are so full of carbohydrates that they qualify as a starch exchange. Make sure you don't limit your selections to these few. Expand your choices to include other vegetables, too.

Take a daily vitamin-mineral supplement. This is especially important if your food choices are not as nutritionally wise this time of month as they normally may be. There will be days when following a diet—even one as accommodating as this one—will be daunting. Anything that requires planning and structure might be stress provoking, which is the last thing you need.

On those days do the following:

- Don't force yourself to eat all the protein, vegetables, fruit, and other foods listed. You're not going to develop malnutrition if you fail to eat a balanced diet for a few days each month. Remember that your primary objective on those days is to feel better and be in control. You can make up any nutritional deficit after you get your period and are feeling better.
- Eat chocolate if that is what you want, as long as it is in low-fat or fat-free form. Here are some chocolate menu suggestions.

Breakfast

1 slice frozen French toast, toasted, spread with 1 tablespoon fat-free chocolate syrup and topped with $^1/_2$ sliced banana.

1 cup fat-free chocolate milk blended with $^1/_2$ cup fat-free cottage cheese and 1 tablespoon chocolate syrup

Equals: 2 protein, 2 starch, 1 fruit

or

1 fat-free brownie halved, spread with 1 cup fat-free sugar-free vanilla yogurt mixed with 1 tablespoon fat-free chocolate syrup

1 glass chocolate milk

Equals: 2 protein, 2 starch

or

chocolate shake (1 cup each of fat-free sugar-free vanilla and chocolate yogurt)

1 chocolate-filled toaster tart

Equals: 2 protein, 1 starch, 1 fat

or

1 cup fat-free pineapple cottage cheese topped with 1 tablespoon chocolate chips or sprinkles

1 fat-free chocolate cookie

Equals: 2 protein, 2 starch

Lunch

1 cup fat-free chocolate pudding (made with fat-free milk) mixed with 1½ cups fat-free chocolate-flavored fat-free breakfast cereal

Equals: 1 protein, 3 starch

or

1 cup fat-free milk mixed with 1 cup diet chocolate soda

1 fat-free chocolate muffin

Equals: 1 protein, 3 starch

or

6 caramel-flavored rice cakes with ½ cup yogurt spread (see p. 155) mixed with chocolate sprinkles and 1 teaspoon honey

Equals: 1 protein, 3 starch

Mid-Afternoon Snack

2 cups chocolate-flavored breakfast cereal mixed with 1 tablespoon fat-free chocolate sauce

Equals: 4 starch

or

1 cup strawberries sprinkled with 2 tablespoons chocolate-
flavored sugar and topped with 1/4 cup chocolate-flavored
nondairy whipped topping
Equals: 2 starch, 1 fruit

Dinner

chocolate roll-ups (3 low-fat flour tortillas lightly toasted,
rolled with 1/4 cup fat-free ricotta mixed with
2 tablespoons chocolate chips and microwaved until
chips melt)
1 cup sliced strawberries
Equals: 3 starch, 1 protein, 1 fruit, 1 fat

or

3 toaster waffles covered with 1/2 cup fat-free chocolate
yogurt, 1/2 banana sliced and topped with 1 tablespoon
fudge sauce.
Equals: 3 starch, 1 protein, 1 fruit

Late-Evening Snack

3 cups plain popcorn with 2 tablespoons of fat-free chocolate
sauce for dipping
Equals: 4 starch

or

2 servings fat-free sugar-free chocolate pudding made with
nonfat milk. Crush 10 malted milk balls and add them
before pudding sets.
Equals: 4 starch

AVOIDING TROUBLE

The mind-over-menstrual-cycle diet is designed to renew serotonin activity as soon as monthly hormonal changes begin to affect it. If you eat the prescribed carbohydrate-rich foods, the enhanced brain serotonin levels and activity that result will quell your urge to overindulge. However, sometimes those hormonal changes will begin to occur while you sleep, with the result that you wake up grumpy and irritable—with an intense yearning for chocolate doughnuts. You may find yourself in the powerful grip of an impulse to devour bags of potato chips, pints of ice cream, or bags of cookies. If this should happen and you end up indulging, here is what you should do: Forget about it. The extra calories from an isolated event aren't going to have a permanent impact on weight loss or maintenance.

But also ask yourself what is going on. Check the calendar. If the date indicates that you are premenstrual, then immediately begin the mind-over-menstrual-cycle diet. Give it a few hours for its serotonin-boosting power to kick in. As soon as it does you will be back in control. And remember to track your menstrual cycle so these mood and appetite changes won't sneak up on you.

Keep these troubleshooting tips in mind.

1. Stock your kitchen with your choice of snacks. Make sure that they are low in fat, and read labels ahead of time so you can relate serving size to calorie and carbohydrate contents.

2. Eat your snack at least one hour before the next meal, don't make it an appetizer.

3. Don't worry or be surprised if your cravings and inability to control your eating vary from month to month. That's absolutely normal.

4. Don't worry too much about nutrition at this time. Take a daily vitamin-mineral supplement that meets the requirements of women.

5. Remember that if you are perimenopausal, that is, entering

the menopausal phase of your life, your PMS may last longer than before. Be prepared.

6. Follow the guidelines for PMS eating control if you are taking hormone replacements, which include a week of progesterone therapy for one week each month; you may feel PMS-like food cravings around the time you take the progesterone.

7. Forget about trying to starve bloating away or preventing it by not drinking enough liquids. Bloating is common and is caused by water retention and also probably by a more sluggish intestinal function at this time. Instead, increase your intake of high-fiber foods or, if necessary, high-fiber supplements.

8. Exercise to sweat off some of the excess water being retained. However, if you are truly uncomfortable, you may not be able to exercise strenuously enough to work up a sweat. This is particularly true when your body feels so tired that your muscles seem heavy. But don't give up on exercise altogether. Gentle exercise, done consistently, will relieve the tiredness, invigorate your muscles, and clear your head. There are many light exercise options. They include low-impact aerobics, walking at a slow speed either outside or indoors on a treadmill, stretching, using either weight machines (for toning) or cardiovascular machines at lower-than-usual intensity, swimming, and water aerobics. If you find your body feels more alive and vigorous after warming up, try to increase the intensity of the exercise so that you work up a sweat. If your PMS lasts for several days or more, it is very important to exercise as often as possible. Otherwise, you might find it hard to start up again once your PMS is over.

9. If coffee or other caffeinated beverages make you jittery, then eliminate them. Caffeine is often a scapegoat for premenstrual ills. If, however, you're feeling spacey and your attention span is nil, then the moderate amounts of caffeine found in a cup of coffee or in a can of cola will perk you up.

10. Chose the nonfat or reduced-fat version of the snack you crave. Reduced-fat or fat-free chocolate and crunchy snack products have become a big business, and new ones are continually being introduced.

Do not starve yourself during the first two or three weeks of your cycle to make up for what you consider overeating during your premenstrual days. Any dietary change that eliminates or markedly reduces sweet and starchy food intake will throw off serotonin balance. If you don't eat a well-balanced, serotonin-sustaining diet (as outlined in Chapter Five) throughout the rest of the month, you will end up suffering from even worse PMS and your appetite will be even more out of control.

Rosemarie was a woman of normal weight who came to see me about what she described as her weight problem. What she really had was a premenstrual eating problem. For about ten out of fourteen days, between ovulation and the onset of her period, she binged. Then, to compensate for her PMS-induced bingeing, she lived on homemade vegetable broth for the first two weeks of her cycle. She would boil carrots, cabbage, string beans, onion, celery, and tomatoes in a big pot of water, discard the cooked vegetables, and drink the broth at mealtimes. That—and a daily vitamin pill—was the extent of her food consumption during this phase of her monthly cycle. By following this severe, not to mention unhealthy, regimen, she was able to control her hunger and cravings until a few days past ovulation. Then, despite her rigid self-discipline, she would inevitably lose the battle against her cravings and, not surprisingly, would start eating everything in sight.

It was easy to understand why she was bingeing. The watery gruel that made up her diet had rid her body of the weight she gained during the second half of her cycle and the serotonin her brain needed. When the added stress of PMS hit her depleted serotonin stores, she was overtaken by such a powerful urge to eat carbohydrates that she was powerless to resist it.

She had been following this pattern for months and was worried—rightfully so—about whether what she was doing was good for her body. I was surprised that she had not developed malnutrition or lost any hair or teeth. She was apprehensive about following my recommendation to increase her calorie intake to normal (for her weight) and to eat carbohydrates at every meal and in at least one snack a day during the first two weeks of her cycle. My suggestions for the premenstrual diet also made her nervous. Compared to what she had been doing, my plan provided what seemed to her enormous quantities of food. Many chronic bingers are reluctant to give up the control over their eating they think a semistarvation diet gives them.

She moved away several months after I first saw her and I lost track of her for a few years. Then, one Sunday morning I was walking my dog and heard my name being called. It was Rosemarie; she had come to Boston for a wedding and was staying at a nearby hotel. She looked great. "I have to tell you that you saved my sanity, as well as my health," she confessed. "I haven't binged *once* since you put me on that special diet. You know, I wasn't going to follow your food plan. It really scared me to think about eating all the foods you told me I could have during the first half of the month, since I was sure that nothing could prevent me from bingeing once I became premenstrual. In fact, when I left your office I almost threw the plan away. But I also knew that I could not go on partially starving myself. Actually, it was my husband who convinced me to try your suggestions. He reminded me that it had been my idea to see you. Why did I bother to do that if I didn't want to change my eating habits? He was right. And so were you. By eating enough carbohydrates early in my cycle, my body really was arming itself against bingeing later on. Of course, I still craved sweets when I was premenstrual. But I could control what I chose to eat and how much. It seems so easy now."

FAMILY, FELLOW WORKERS, AND FRIENDS

Your family should be told ahead of time that you may be eating what is, to them, an odd assortment of foods on some days and that this is an important part of your diet. If possible, you want to avoid being teased about your eating. Let people know that these apparent eccentricities are in fact part of a carefully thought-out strategy.

You should also make sure that family members understand that when you are premenstrual you would prefer not to be confronted by arguments, major decisions, or the need to act as mediator.

Of course, work associates do not need to know about the ups and downs of your monthly moods. But when possible, try to avoid scheduling complicated work assignments, travel obligations, or demanding meetings on those days when you know you may not be as sharp, patient, or focused as usual. A lot of these things won't be under your control, no matter how carefully you plan, so food will be your best ally at these times. If anyone asks why you are eating chocolate cupcakes and marshmallows at eleven in the morning or drinking hot chocolate instead of your usual tea in the afternoon, try telling them the Aztecs founded an entire civilization while drinking chocolate; think what it could do for *you.*

Social obligations, of course, take planning. If possible, I advise you to avoid dinner parties—both going to and giving them. If you must go, arm yourself beforehand and have that all-important snack before you leave the house, and take another one in your purse for after dinner (so you can skip dessert and eat what will make you feel better). If, on the other hand, you are forced to have people over, try an all low-fat chocolate dessert buffet. Your guests will thank you for it and you will have the foods you need in the comfort of your own home.

A LAST WORD

For many women, finding private time in order to enjoy the foods they are craving and the peace and rest their bodies are demanding is extremely difficult. That time, however, is crucial.

Be good to yourself when you are premenstrual. You can enhance the stress-relieving properties of the diet by giving yourself time to enjoy pleasures you usually put on the back burner. If there is an activity you like but keep putting off because of lack of time or money, or because you feel guilty about being self-indulgent, try to do it when you are premenstrual. Get that overdue haircut. If you can afford to do so, get a facial, a massage, or a manicure. Spend a half hour checking out hair ornaments and makeup. Spritz yourself with a new perfume. Buy a pair of inexpensive earrings. (Forget about trying on clothes: They won't fit right.) Go to a local plant nursery and check out the new shipment of seedlings. Rent a video and watch it when no one else is around. Hire a baby-sitter and go to a movie with a friend. (See a sad one and have a good cry if you want to.)

Yes, you know that this time will pass—and by following the diet, you'll make sure it won't be one that you'll have to dread anymore.

CHAPTER EIGHT

Diets for All Seasons

Are you one of those people who begin to gain weight every fall as soon as the leaves hit the ground? When the days grow darker, cloudy, and snowy, and sunlight becomes a vague memory, do you invariably start to eat and sleep a lot more?

Until the mid-1980s no one had identified winter depression as a syndrome, nor understood that its components included extreme tiredness, irritability, and ineffectiveness. However, it *was* taken for granted that cabin fever would strike as soon as the temperature dipped below freezing, the snow and ice piled up, and the inevitable strains of flu raced through schoolrooms and office buildings. Of course we all feel depressed and lethargic during the winter. Who doesn't?

It was also assumed that many people would end the winter months fatter than before, sort of a reverse hibernation. "You need to add a layer of fat for insulation" was the accepted reason for the five- or ten-pound weight gain of winter. Oddly enough, no one seemed to question the logic of this. Heated homes, offices, and cars, thermal underwear, down-filled coats, and heavy boots did their jobs extremely well. Nevertheless, winter and weight gain went hand in hand, as inevitable as tax returns in

April. There seemed to be nothing to do about it except bear it (no pun intended).

In 1984 a group of researchers at the National Institutes of Health became interested in a group of people who were depressed in the winter but felt fine if they journeyed south, where the climate was warmer and the sun rose earlier and set later than up north. In an experiment designed to determine whether it was the rise in temperature or the longer period of daylight that was responsible for the depression relief, the researchers asked volunteers to sit in front of a box containing between four and six very bright fluorescent lights for one to two hours in the morning and again in the evening.

The researchers found the early morning exposure to light had a dramatic effect on lifting the volunteers' depression. However, the evening exposure was less helpful. They also discovered that in order to be effective, light had to enter the subjects' eyes; when their eyes were covered and only their skin was exposed, the volunteers' moods did not improve. On the basis of this and other similar experiments, the NIH researchers eventually named and described a new type of depressive disorder: seasonal affective disorder (SAD). People who suffer from SAD tend to experience its symptoms yearly. It appears to be triggered by the steady decrease in the hours of daylight that begins mid-fall and lasts until mid-spring. The first symptoms are usually profound fatigue accompanied by a compelling urge to eat excessive amounts of sweet and starchy foods. As the days grow shorter, other symptoms appear. Depression; a nearly uncontrollable need to sleep; and lack of interest in work, family, and social activities define the fully developed syndrome.

Untreated, the combination of eating and sleeping more and moving less causes an inevitable weight gain. SAD sufferers can put on up to fifty pounds over a six-month period. Day after day, week after week, the person with SAD wants to do only two things: eat and sleep.

Years ago I had a client who was a typical SAD sufferer. When I attempted to learn how she managed her life during the long, dark New England winters, she told me that she did nothing after work except go to bed. "I get into my nightgown and robe about 4 P.M. Then I stockpile boxes of cookies, bags of chips, and cans of soda on the floor near my bed. I get under the covers, reading and eating until about 7 P.M. Then I go to sleep." Her weekends weren't much different. She crawled out of bed on Saturday morning and made it to a nearby bake shop, where she stocked up on muffins and pastries. On the way home she bought some magazines. At home she got back into bed and stayed there pretty much full-time until Monday morning. Not surprisingly, she gained about forty-five pounds every winter.

However, you don't have to experience a severe case of SAD to suffer winter weight gain. In the last few years additional research has revealed that many people experience a milder version of SAD. It has been given the tongue-twisting name of subsyndromal SAD; I prefer to call it winter weight gain. It, too, is defined as sort of a reverse semihibernation: You end the winter heavier than you were in the fall. Although you do not suffer from the extreme depression or excessive sleepiness of SAD, you feel tired, apathetic, and hungry for carbohydrates all the time, a condition that is with you from the time you wake up in the morning until the time you go to sleep. Your life is put on hold during these months; what limited energy you have is focused on having enough carbohydrates to eat, and clean pajamas to eat in.

Thankfully, spring and summer bring relief from apathy, tiredness, and uncontrolled eating. The long days of late spring and summer represent the other swing of the depressed mood–overeating pendulum. During these seasons SAD sufferers are catapulted into a mood characterized by surges of energy and euphoria. It is easy for them to lose weight at this time of year because their food cravings are gone and they no longer feel the constant need to eat. Since they are also likely to be physically active thanks to their high energy, the potential for weight loss is further increased. Now is the perfect time for dieting—when appetite is normal and controllable, and exercising is pleasurable.

One client told me that she always knew she had entered her summer high when she could walk past her freezer and forget the ice cream there. All winter she had to maintain a large supply of it because she could not get through an evening without eating at least a pint. "But once the days get long," she told me, "the switch in my head that constantly nagged me to eat shuts itself off. I realized the other day that the ice cream I bought in May is untouched. And here it is, the middle of July."

WHY MANY PEOPLE CAN'T KEEP WEIGHT OFF

I believe these seasonal swings in mood and eating pattern are a major reason why numerous people can't control their eating and weight during the winter. And yet, the same people who go completely out of control during the winter can be quite disciplined the rest of the year. If you're one of them, you're familiar with the annual rites. Every spring you decide to go on a diet, and you know from past experience that it will work. Now it seems easy to count calories, to weigh and measure food, to say no to rich desserts. Every day you walk, bike, or go to the gym. You say to yourself, "This is great. I feel good; I'm losing weight at a steady pace; exercise—no problem. This time I know I'm not going to gain back any weight. I've finally learned to control my cravings and impulsive overeating. This time it's for keeps." Then November rolls around with its short overcast days and long nights, and once again you lose it all. Willpower vanishes, and the idea of exercise becomes unthinkable. You find yourself packing in the macaroni and cheese, French fries, pizza, and chocolate cake all day long, then curling up in bed for whatever remains of your waking hours. You say, "Tomorrow—I'll get back on track." But you don't. And that weight comes back.

If you have joined a regular weight-loss group or one that provides nutritional counseling, you may feel even worse. Because winter weight-gain disorder is usually not recognized by these programs, you may find yourself berated for failing to abide by the rules of behavior modification or recommendations on sensible eating patterns and/or daily exercise. And after repeatedly spending a lot of time and money on spring-summer diet programs, you just give up. What is the sense, you might think, of trying to lose weight every summer if it's just going to be packed on again several months later? Why buy clothes that will only fit until the end of September? Why spend hard-earned money for a health club membership that won't be used once the sun starts setting at 5 P.M.?

With all this in mind, please believe that giving up is not the answer—if only because it's too dangerous. Even a small weight gain of five to ten pounds every winter will eventually add up to a total gain so high that you can be at risk for the medical disorders associated with obesity. Conventional methods are not going to address this problem. If they could, you would not be thirty or more pounds heavier today than you were ten years ago, even though you have been dieting for at least eight of those ten years.

Angry and frustrated with yourself, you may think that the fault lies in your lack of willpower and self-control. It doesn't. You are another victim of winter weight gain. SAD and winter depression are textbook examples of a physiological stress that you cannot prevent any more than you can prevent the seasons from changing.

My colleagues and I have studied the problem of winter weight gain since the late 1980s. The research we have done points toward an easy and effective solution—a two-part diet. During the winter you follow part one, a 2,000–plus calorie "Winter Weight-Maintenance" plan. Instead of fighting winter carbohydrate craving, you'll learn how to use carbohydrate foods therapeutically to control overeating, overcome winter blues, and even boost your energy levels. During the rest of the year you can go on the under–1,200 calorie "Spring-Summer Slim-Down" regimen—and do just that.

THE SOLUTION: THE SEROTONIN CONNECTION

The two-part diet is based on what our research has shown us about seasonal variations in brain serotonin activity in those people who suffer from regular winter weight gain. The dark days of winter somehow depress their serotonin production, with the result that they eat more and exercise less. Winter darkness may also disturb the normal rhythm of another brain chemical, melatonin, which is usually absent from the blood during the day. It's not clear what role melatonin plays in SAD. The best explanation so far is that light really does alter melatonin, and this change, in turn, affects serotonin. While the mechanisms behind these brain changes are not yet known, what we do know for certain is that if serotonin activity can be increased, SAD symptoms will decrease.

One means of manipulating serotonin activity is via drugs specifically developed for that purpose. In the late 1980s Dr. Dermot O'Rourke and I treated patients suffering from SAD with dexfenfluramine to see whether this drug might prevent weight gain during the winter months. For three years we conducted studies during the late fall and winter, always being careful to end the studies by early March, since we wanted to make sure the drug was responsible for reducing carbohydrate cravings, and not the increased hours of daylight that begin in early spring.

We found the drug was extremely effective in halting overeating, promoting weight loss, and relieving all the mood changes associated with SAD. Recent studies using drugs like Prozac, Zoloft, and other antidepressants that also affect serotonin have confirmed that serotonin is a key element in SAD.

As was discussed in Chapter Two, where I described my research on food and mood, eating low-fat, high-carbohydrate foods is another way of increasing serotonin activity and thereby promoting emotional well-being and reducing carbohydrate cravings. Dr. Norman Rosenthal, at the NIH, one of the medical researchers who discovered SAD, has done some more recent studies showing that this is so. Borrowing the techniques we used at MIT in which we measured the moods of volunteers both before and after eating carbohydrates, he fed his volunteers special crackers made for him at our Clinical Research Center.

There was a dramatic improvement in the levels of depression, anger, fatigue, and tension in people with SAD after they ate high-carbohydrate meals (but not after protein meals).

So nature, in her wisdom, has provided us with an easy and convenient way of dealing with the short, dark days of winter: food. Unfortunately, if food is to be used therapeutically to combat SAD, relatively large doses of sweet and starchy carbohydrates will need to be taken frequently. Frankly, trying to go on a weight-loss diet this time of year has as much chance of success as attempting to prevent the leaves from falling. But even if you can't lose weight, you can prevent yourself from gaining it with the winter weight-maintenance diet. Then, if you want to lose weight, you can start following the spring-summer slim-down diet as soon as the hours of sunlight are longer than the hours of darkness. If you begin the spring-summer slim-down when the clocks change from standard to daylight saving time and continue until they change back, you will have six months of weight-loss time.

THE MAINTENANCE PLAN

How the Plan Works

Since serotonin is the key to relieving SAD, the winter weight-stabilizing plan makes sure you get a dose of serotonin-promoting carbohydrates every time you need one, beginning after breakfast and ending before you go to sleep. All the meals and snacks after breakfast are carefully designed to provide enough carbohydrates to activate the insulin-tryptophan-serotonin connection, and their timing is based on our knowledge that the effect on serotonin starts to fade within about three hours after eating the carbohydrates.

Breakfast is the only meal that contains a substantial amount of protein. Your body requires protein to maintain optimum health, and you must eat the lion's share of your protein separately from your carbohydrates. And since your winter-induced carbohydrate cravings only intensify as the day goes on, breakfast is probably your last chance to eat protein without threatening to throw your whole serotonin balance out of whack. It's a brief window of opportunity for protein, and it must be taken advantage of, even if you awake already longing for carbohydrates.

If you cannot bear the thought of swallowing eggs or cottage cheese at 7 A.M. on a February morning, try this: Buy a diet powder, double the amount specified for a meal, and add it to your juice or milk. That way you will drink the required amount of protein. Or blend your own drink using cottage cheese (try a fruit-flavored variety), milk, a banana, and a squirt of low-fat chocolate syrup.

SAMPLE MAINTENANCE MENUS

Breakfast Exchanges

3 protein (24 grams)
3 starch (45 grams)
1 fruit (15 grams)
total calories: 510

Sample Breakfasts

2 scrambled eggs with 2 slices fat-free cheese (cooked with
    nonstick spray)
1 English muffin (sandwich-size) with 1 teaspoon jelly
1 orange
Equals: 3 protein, 3 starch, 1 fruit

or

baked apple (prepare the day before) on bed of cinnamon-
    sugar-flavored fat-free cottage cheese (1½ cups cottage
    cheese plus 2 teaspoons sugar)
2 slices raisin toast
Equals: 3 protein, 3 starch, 1 fruit

or

2 toaster waffles
1 tablespoon pancake syrup
2 slices smoked turkey
2 slices fat-free cheese
1 6-ounce glass orange juice
Equals: 3 protein, 2 carbohydrate, 1 fruit, 1 "free"

or

$1^1/_2$ cups pineapple cottage cheese (fat-free)
1 fat-free bran muffin with 1 tablespoon apple butter
6 ounces diet cranberry juice
Equals: 3 protein, 3 carbohydrate, 1 fruit

Mid-Morning Snack

45 grams of carbohydrate

Lunch Exchanges

2 protein (16 grams)
3 starch (45 grams)
2 vegetable (10 grams)
1 fat (5 grams)
total calories: 475

Sample Lunches

2 ounces lean roast beef sliced very thin
2 slices rye bread
$^1/_2$ cup baked potato chips
mustard
1 cup coleslaw with fat-free dressing and 3 chopped black olives
1 pear (instead of additional starch exchange)
Equals: 2 protein, 3 starch, 2 vegetable, 1 fruit

or

1 cup microwaveable vegetables and noodle soup
1 sandwich consisting of 2 ounces mock seafood salad made
    with fat-free mayonnaise
1 tangerine
1 cup carrot slices and cucumber slices
Equals: 2 protein, 3 starch, 1 vegetable, 1 fruit

or

1$^1/_2$ cups steamed rice
2 ounces stir-fried chicken
1 cup stir-fried vegetables (onions, peppers, mushrooms,
    tomatoes)
1 apple
Equals: 2 protein, 3 starch, 2 vegetable, 1 fruit

Mid-Afternoon Snack

45 grams of carbohydrate

Dinner Exchanges

1 protein (8 grams)
3 starch (45 grams)
2 vegetable (10 grams)
1 fruit (15 grams)
1 fat (5 grams)
total calories: 465

Sample Dinners

corn soup*
1 cup steamed spinach

*recipe on page 147

1 pear
Equals: 1 protein, 3 starch, 2 vegetable, 1 fruit, 1 fat

or

country pea soup*
1 fruit
Equals: 1 protein, 3 starch, 2 vegetable, 1 fruit

or

American chop suey[†]
1 cup raw spinach salad with fat-free dressing and 1 teaspoon
    soy "bacon bits"
1 orange
Equals: 1 protein, 3 starch, 2 vegetable, 1 fruit, 1 fat, 1 "free"

or

creamy garlic spaghetti[††]
2 cups salad consisting of romaine lettuce and 1 tablespoon
    fat-free dressing
1 sliced apple
Equals: 1 protein, 3 starch, 2 vegetable, 1 fruit, 1 "free"

Mid-Evening Snack

1 starch (15 grams)
1 fruit (15 grams)
total calories: 140

*recipe on page 147
[†]recipe on page 148
[††]recipe on page 148

RECIPES

Corn Soup

Serves 1

> 1 medium onion, sliced thin
> $1/2$ cup sweet red pepper, diced
> 1 teaspoon olive oil
> 2 medium potatoes, chopped
> 1 cube of chicken or vegetable bouillon
> 1 cup boiling water
> 1 teaspoon cornstarch
> 1 cup fat-free milk
> 1 teaspoon salt
> $1/4$ teaspoon pepper
> 6 ounces niblet corn
> 1 teaspoon curry powder (optional)

Cook onions and pepper in saucepan coated with 1 teaspoon olive oil. Add chopped potatoes and cook until tender. Dissolve bouillon cube in boiling water. Add cornstarch to $1/4$ cup of fat-free milk, stir until smooth, and add to potato/vegetable mixture. Add bouillon. Cook until smooth and thick. Add remaining milk, salt, pepper, corn, and curry powder. Simmer fifteen minutes.

Country Pea Soup

Serves 8

> 1 pound yellow peas
> 8 cups boiling water
> 4 cups tomato juice
> ham bone with 4 ounces meat, or smoked turkey. If you

want to keep it vegetarian, add 4 vegetarian sausages instead, broken in small fragments
1 1/2 cups potato, diced
1 cup onion, diced
2 cups carrots, diced
1 small bay leaf
salt and pepper to taste

Wash peas. Put water and tomato juice in large kettle. Bring to a boil, turn down heat, cover tightly, and simmer until peas are soft, about forty-five minutes. Add ham bone and all remaining ingredients. Cover and simmer until vegetables are tender, about forty-five minutes. Discard ham bone and bay leaf. Taste and adjust seasoning. For a main dish, eat two servings.

American Chop Suey

2 cups of elbow macaroni, cooked
1 cup meatless tomato sauce
1 ounce lean beef, cooked
1/2 cup sautéed mushrooms
1 teaspoon olive oil

Sauté mushrooms in olive oil. After mushrooms are firm, add lean beef and cook until brown. Pour in tomato sauce, cook together for 20 minutes and pour over cooked macaroni.

Creamy Garlic Spaghetti

Serves 2

4 ounces (uncooked weight) spaghetti
2 cloves garlic, minced
2 teaspoons olive oil
4 ounces fat-free ricotta cheese

oregano and basil to taste
¹/₄ cup Parmesan cheese, grated

Cook spaghetti. Sauté garlic in olive oil. Toss drained spaghetti with ricotta cheese, oregano, basil, and garlic olive oil. Sprinkle with Parmesan cheese.

AVOIDING TROUBLE

1. Eat as little fat as you can tolerate in order to avoid gaining weight. *Remember: This is a weight-maintenance diet.* The only way you will be able both to keep your calorie intake under control and to eat as many carbohydrates as you will be craving is to eat them with as little fat as possible.

2. Take a vitamin-mineral supplement every day. If you are not going to be eating at least 1¹/₂ to 2 cups of dairy products a day, take a calcium supplement. If you are premenopausal you need eight hundred milligrams a day; if you have entered menopause you require one thousand milligrams of calcium daily.

3. Make sure you eat enough fiber. If you are not eating a substantial amount of fruit and vegetables (and you should be), make sure you eat a high-fiber cereal like bran or take a high-fiber drink or pill daily.

4. Drink plenty of liquids. Office and home heating systems can be as dehydrating as the summer sun.

5. Avoid alcohol. Winter weight gain disorder and SAD are known to increase alcohol intake. Alcohol, in addition to its other effects, is notorious for adding pounds.

6. Force yourself to shop for food regularly and plan your shopping with a list. Otherwise, you will find yourself steering your cart down the supermarket aisles that are stocked with high-fat ice cream, cookies, and snack foods. These are not the foods that will help you maintain your weight—or your serotonin levels. To make buying the right foods easier, make a list around the end of October of the basic high-nutrient foods you intend to eat all winter long. Type or print it out, and make a copy to carry in

your wallet at all times. When you go food shopping, take out the list and follow it. Do not make bargains with yourself, the kind that say, "I will buy one pint of regular ice cream for every pint of fat-free frozen yogurt."

Here's a sample weekly shopping list:

7 containers of fat-free, 100-calorie-per-serving yogurt
1 quart fat-free pineapple cottage cheese
1 quart 1 percent or 2 percent milk
1 box high-fiber cereal
1 box sweet, low-fat cereal
1 quart orange juice
6 bananas
3 oranges
2 boxes frozen broccoli
1 box frozen string beans
1 box frozen squash
1 box frozen peas
1 small bunch carrots (every other week)
7 flip-top cans of tuna in water, 3 ounces each
$1/2$ pound of cooked sliced chicken or turkey
$1/2$ dozen eggs
1 pound ground turkey
1 package turkey sausage
1 package boneless, skinless chicken breasts
1 package English muffins
1 package fresh or dried pasta
1 box rice (Flavored rice makes a fast dinner. Use only half
    the spice mix provided in order to keep down salt intake.)
3 cans baked beans, 16 ounces each
1 box instant mashed potatoes
3 to 4 containers of dried or canned soup
coffee/tea/diet soft drinks/low-fat hot chocolate mix
cooking oil/spices/herbs, etc., as needed

Snacks do not require a list, since you are on your own to pick what you like (see page 92 for suggestions).

Don't let your boxes of frozen vegetables and packages of skinless chicken breasts and ground turkey burgers hibernate in your freezer. Eat them.

7. Pay attention to portion sizes. The plan provides ample calories and substantial—but not unrestricted—amounts of carbohydrates. If you follow the portion sizes you will not gain weight.

8. Be sure to exercise. Yes, the state of semihibernation is incompatible with physical activity. However, without exercise your muscles, the body's biggest calorie users, will decrease; summer dieting will be that much harder. Here are some ideas for winter exercise:

- Walk briskly through a shopping mall two or three times a week with a friend.
- Go bowling. It's an indoor sport, brightly lit, and fun. (If you are afraid that it's too strenuous, remember that you can always sit down after your turn.)
- Play Ping-Pong. Bending and stretching to retrieve and return the ball will keep you limber; the running will work your heart.
- Go to a pool. Either swim or use one of those devices that tether you to a wall of the pool, allowing you to walk or do exercises in the water. That way you can get a good workout without muscle strain. The wet warmth of an indoor pool is often a welcome relief from the skin-cracking dryness of most heated indoor spaces. Even if you just walk back and forth in the water, you will be hydrating your body and doing it some good.
- Use weight-training machines. Since you probably won't *want* to go to a health club or Y, find someone who is committed to dragging you there. Getting a workout buddy is a great way of getting yourself out the door. If this is your first time—or your first time in a long while—ask a trainer to help you figure out how to use the machines. They can be intimidating to a beginner, and they can also cause muscle strains and pulls if you don't know the proper settings to use for

weight and placement adjustments. But after a few tries you'll know what you need to know and will start to feel comfortable with the machines.

Yes, you will find it hard to motivate yourself in the winter; you feel so much more tired that time of year. But I can promise you that, after you exercise, you will be more energetic and awake.

A friend of mine and her husband used to drag themselves to a health club after work in the winter. They both felt so exhausted they didn't have the energy to talk to each other on the way. But they had made a commitment to work out together, and neither one wanted to be called "wimp." "It was amazing to see the transformation that came over us after we had finished our workouts," she told me. "Sure, my body was tired from the exercise and my muscles ached a bit. But my head became clear, I could talk again, and I felt the evening ahead was something to look forward to rather than just something to be gotten through before going to sleep."

The maintenance plan should make you feel less depressed and more lively. But it will not substitute for the wonderfully long days of June and July. Nor, in the middle of February, will it have the same effect as lying on a beach where it is blissfully warm. It will, however, furnish you with frequent therapeutic doses of carbohydrates that will guarantee peak serotonin function. And you may find that your winter blues diminish even if they don't disappear.

Another thing you might consider trying is light therapy. Although it has no effect on appetite, carbohydrate cravings, or winter weight gain, many psychologists and psychiatrists—and even a few physicians—currently recommend this as a therapy for SAD-related depression. The therapy consists of exposure to intense artificial light of a particular spectrum and wavelength that mimics the early morning light of late spring and summer. It is delivered by a large metal box fitted with special fluorescent lightbulbs. There are at least a dozen companies in this country that manufacture these light boxes. Many psychiatrists know about their employment against depression. The light boxes must be used daily for at least thirty minutes or longer in the early morning. If more than two or three days are skipped, SAD symptoms will return.

SPRING-SUMMER SLIM-DOWN PLAN

At last, the clocks have been pushed forward, the buds are on the trees, and it's time to slim down. As the days grow longer your mental and physical energy will begin to return to normal. Your need to eat excessive amounts of carbohydrates will start to diminish, because the longer hours of daylight have returned serotonin activity to normal. By the time you decide to take the winter clothes to the cleaner you will find yourself ready, willing, and able to throw the winter's crackers, cookies, cakes, and cereals to the returning birds.

The spring-summer slim-down plan harnesses your now-powered-up eating control, along with your body's urge for physical activity and your recharged commitment to losing weight. You will lose that weight easily and effortlessly.

How the Plan Works

Notice that you are allowed relatively few carbohydrate-rich foods on this plan, compared to its winter counterpart. Also, portion sizes have been cut back and snacks have been eliminated. If you still want to nibble on something during your usual snacking times, put aside some fruit, fat-free dairy products, or vegetables from your regular meals and have them later. If you have a taste for something cold and sweet, have an Italian ice, a watermelon slush, a frozen fruit-juice bar, or a low-fat frozen fudge pop. These frozen treats are incredibly refreshing on a hot day. Do reserve them for the dog days of summer, though, and not as a daily snack—their calories add up.

Summertime is on your side, providing a huge variety of low-calorie fruits and vegetables that minimize your feelings of deprivation. Roasted vegetables and portobello mushrooms prepared on a barbecue grill are delicious, low-calorie alternatives to hamburgers and hot dogs. Corn on the cob, fresh blueberries, poached salmon, boiled lobster, steamed clams, cold beet or cucumber soup, or vegetables eaten right from the garden all make summer dieting a lot easier. As long as you don't add fat you can enjoy all the delicacies of summer.

Because vegetables are low in calories and are available in such a large variety, they can enhance the taste and texture of all your meals and fill you up without exceeding your calorie limitations. So experiment with new ways of preparing them or incorporating them into your entrees. Steamed or roasted vegetables can be marinated, chilled, and served as appetizers or tossed with cooked rice or pasta. Red and green cabbage can be shredded and mixed with carrots, onions, dill, red and green peppers, fresh corn, and tuna or cooked, diced chicken for a filling and colorful low-calorie meal. Chop fresh tomatoes with spring onions, basil, or oregano for a quick no-cook spaghetti sauce. Mix sliced cucumbers and dill with plain fat-free yogurt for a soothing side dish or as a dressing for cold poached fish. Soups can be fast and simple; use a dried soup mix as a base and add a handful of fresh or frozen vegetables. And don't overlook nutrient-dense leafy green vegetables. Chop kale with onion, garlic, and low-fat turkey or vegetarian sausage, cook the mixture in chicken broth, splash it with vinegar, and enjoy a main course. A smooth spinach soup can be created in minutes. Just steam the greens and puree them in a blender with plain fat-free yogurt or buttermilk. Sprinkle with nutmeg and serve. Long lettuce leaves can be wrapped around a mixture of cold rice, leftover chicken or beef, red peppers, onion, and fat-free Italian salad dressing for a low-calorie roll-up. Don't forget potato salad: Mix boiled and cooled spuds with chopped carrots, tomatoes, cucumbers, pickles, and red pepper, and bind with fat-free mayonnaise. And the robust meaty taste of mushrooms can serve as an excellent addition to sauces or soups. If your acquaintance with vegetables is limited to boxes of frozen peas and carrots, treat yourself to a vegetarian cook-book. There are endless numbers of great-tasting dishes you can learn to make.

Unless you coat vegetables with high-fat ingredients, you can enjoy large portions without going over your calorie limit. And you will not only feel healthy, you'll be filled up as well.

Continue to take your daily vitamin-mineral supplement as insurance against those days when you may not eat as well as you intended. Add a calcium supplement if your gender, age, and food choices require that you do so.

MENU SUGGESTIONS FOR SPRING-SUMMER SLIM-DOWN DIET

Breakfast Exchanges

1 protein (8 grams)
1 starch (15 grams)
1 fruit (15 grams)
total calories: 210

Sample Breakfasts

Banana shake made with 8 ounces fat-free milk and 1 banana
(substitute for starch exchange)
Equals: 1 protein, 1 fruit, 1 starch

or

$1/2$ cinnamon raisin bagel spread with $1/2$ cup vanilla-flavored yogurt spread (make by draining 1 cup yogurt through cheesecloth overnight)
1 orange
Equals: 1 protein, 1 starch, 1 fruit

or

$^3/_4$ cup raisin bran cereal
8 ounces fat-free milk
$^1/_2$ cup blueberries
Equals: 1 protein, 1 starch, 1 fruit

Lunch Exchanges

2 protein (16 grams)
2 starch (30 grams)
2 vegetable (10 grams)
total calories: 350

Sample Lunch

2 ounces turkey luncheon meat
1 thin slice (fat-free) Swiss cheese
2 thin slices rye bread
mustard
2 cups salad with 1 chopped carrot and 1 sliced sweet red
    pepper
Equals: 2 protein, 2 starch, 2 vegetable

or

2 ounces water-packed tuna mixed with $^1/_2$ chopped
    cucumber, 2 stalks celery, 1 teaspoon chopped onion,
    $^1/_2$ cup chopped red pepper, served on green leafy lettuce
    bed with 1 tomato
1 tablespoon fat-free mayonnaise
4 cheese-flavored rice cakes
Equals: 2 protein, 2 starch, 1 vegetable

or

1 vegetarian burger
1 hamburger bun
1 thin slice onion

pickle relish (1 teaspoon)

2 cups chopped red cabbage mixed with 1 tablespoon fat-free coleslaw dressing

Equals: 2 protein, 2 starch, 2 vegetable

Dinner Exchanges

3 protein (24 grams)
2 starch (30 grams)
2 vegetable (10 grams)
1 fruit (15 grams)
1 fat (5 grams)
total calories: 525

Sample Dinners

3 ounces fish drizzled with 1 teaspoon olive oil baked with sauce of one chopped tomato, $^1/_2$ onion, 1 red pepper, 1 cup mushrooms, Italian seasoning

1 cup cooked rice

1 pear

Equals: 3 protein, 2 starch, 2 vegetable, 1 fruit, 1 fat

or

3 ounces very lean beef, sliced thin

stir-fry with 1 green pepper, 1 red pepper, 1 cup mushrooms, 1 onion, 1 garlic clove, 1 teaspoon olive oil

add $^1/_2$ cup tomato sauce

ladle over 1 cup cooked noodles

1 wedge watermelon

Equals: 3 protein, 2 starch, 2 vegetable, 1 fruit, 1 fat

or

3 ounces (raw) chicken breast

baked with orange, mustard, honey sauce (make sauce by

mixing $1/4$ cup orange juice, 1 teaspoon mustard, 1 teaspoon honey. Serve with orange slices from $1/2$ orange and sprinkle with 1 teaspoon sliced almonds)
1 small or half large baked sweet potato
1 cup steamed broccoli
Equals: 3 protein, 2 starch, 2 vegetable, 1 fruit, 1 fat

Snack

Eat a fat-free sweet or starch snack once a day—either late afternoon or mid-evening. It should contain 45 grams of carbohydrate and no more than 210 calories.

RECIPES

Wintertime Pasta

Slightly higher in fat than some, but oh, so comforting when those winter winds begin to blow.

Serves 4

12 ounces fresh pasta
1 tablespoon unsalted butter
4 cloves garlic, crushed
2 tablespoons fresh sage leaves, chopped (use dried if fresh not available; reduce amount to $1/2$ teaspoon)
2 ounces prosciutto, cut into thin shreds
$1/4$ cup black olives, pitted
freshly ground black pepper
2 tablespoons low-fat Parmesan cheese

Cook the pasta according to package directions. Meanwhile, heat the butter in a small saucepan with the garlic and sage until warm.

Toss the pasta with the aromatic butter mixture; add prosciutto and olives. Sprinkle with cheese.

A salad of leafy lettuce, spinach, and sliced mushrooms is a good accompaniment.

Skelk

A traditional Irish dish, sure to warm your heart. If you have a fat exchange to spare, drizzle with a teaspoon of melted butter.

Serves 6

6 large, all-purpose potatoes, peeled, quartered, and cut into
    chunks
10 scallions, sliced thin, including tops
$1/2$ cup evaporated skim milk
salt and pepper and dill to taste

Put the potatoes in a large saucepan with water to cover. Bring to a boil and cook over medium heat until tender, approximately twenty minutes. Meanwhile, wilt the scallions in the milk in a small saucepan over medium heat, about five minutes. Mash the potatoes thoroughly, add the scallions and milk, and season generously with salt, pepper and a tablespoon of chopped dill. A salad of sliced tomatoes, chopped red onions, a dash of balsamic vinegar and 1 teaspoon of olive oil goes well with this dish.

Warm Broccoli Salad

A wonderful wintertime salad, but good enough for any season. Roasted red peppers are now found in jars and are available at specialty and food shops everywhere.

Serves 2

1 bunch fresh broccoli, broken into florets
2 cloves garlic, crushed
1 tablespoon olive oil
$1/_3$ cup roasted red peppers or canned pimiento, cut into bite-sized pieces
10 small black or niçoise-type olives
1 tablespoon balsamic vinegar
1 tablespoon fresh basil or parsley, chopped
salt and pepper to taste

Stir fry the broccoli and garlic together in olive oil until tender. Add a tablespoon or two of water and the red peppers. Cover the pan and allow to steam three minutes. Toss together with the remaining ingredients and serve.

Save leftover salad and mix with cooked chicken or lean beef strips for another meal.

Grilled Summer Chicken

Perfect lightweight backyard barbecue.

Serves 4

1 pound boneless, skinless chicken breasts
$1/_2$ cup fat-free mayonnaise
2 tablespoons honey
3 tablespoons strong, Dijon-type mustard
2 tablespoons apple cider vinegar
1 teaspoon hot sauce, or to taste
2 cloves garlic, crushed

Cut the chicken into serving-sized pieces; rinse and pat dry. Combine remaining ingredients and pour over the chicken breasts. Allow to marinate in the refrigerator for at least three hours. Grill on an electric, gas, or charcoal grill until very tender, approximately five to seven minutes on each side.

If you live all year in a warm climate, do not wait for the summer to make this.

Summertime Pasta Salad

Serves 1 as a meal or 3 to 4 as a side dish

1 1/2 cups bowtie pasta, uncooked
1/2 cup plain, fat-free yogurt
1 tablespoon Dijon-type mustard
1/2 teaspoon salt
2 green onions, chopped, including tops
1 large clove garlic, crushed
3 or 4 plum tomatoes, cut into bite-sized pieces
1 or 2 jalapeño peppers (optional)

Cook the pasta according to package directions; rinse and chill slightly. Toss with remaining ingredients, cover, and refrigerate two hours before serving.

Nonfat Balsamic Vinaigrette

Summer is indeed the salad season, and this wonderful rich-tasting accompaniment will guarantee that your salads will never get dull.

1/4 cup balsamic vinegar
3 tablespoons fat-free mayonnaise
3 tablespoons orange juice
3 tablespoons water
2 cloves garlic, crushed
1 teaspoon fresh oregano, or 1/4 teaspoon dried
1 tablespoon chopped fresh basil, or 1 teaspoon dried
1/4 teaspoon sugar
salt and pepper to taste

Whisk all ingredients together. Cover tightly and refrigerate before use.

AVOIDING TROUBLE

1. Watch your portion sizes (except vegetables, where you should feel free to exceed recommendations if that's what you need to fill you up). During the first week on the diet, make sure that you are paying attention to the size of the protein servings. Do not overeat. This is very important: Your appetite for protein will be much greater now than it was during the fall and winter.

2. Watch your alcohol intake. Barbecues, boat trips, vacations are all occasions for social drinking. Since your calorie intake has to be controlled, be sure that alcoholic beverages don't push you over your limit. To minimize alcohol consumption, add a splash of white wine to a glass of seltzer, or ask for a light beer and sip very slowly.

3. Learn how to make vegetables part of the main course. Portobello mushrooms, for instance, are a tasty low-calorie substitute for meat when roasted or broiled. Adding hefty portions of vegetables to dishes that contain lesser quantities of meat allows you to increase serving sizes without upping caloric intake.

4. Be careful while on vacation. You may wish to go off your diet to allow yourself to indulge in those special foods you only have away from home. If the Fourth of July or some other special occasion is not complete without fried clams or a baked stuffed lobster or a berry pie topped with vanilla ice cream or whatever—then go ahead: Enjoy the day. You can minimize some of the calorie overload by eating only until you are full. And make sure that prior to and following that special meal you are careful about the other food choices of the day.

5. Do not skip the snack. You must eat it daily to ensure adequate serotonin production otherwise you may experience

a deficit in brain serotonin levels that will leave you vulnerable to emotional overeating when the summer diet ends (see Chapter Eleven).

6. Beware of summertime stress. Anyone who has taken a trip with children or has arrived at a longed-for destination only to encounter the worst weather in one hundred years knows summer has its share of stress. And of course the same daily stresses that are present the rest of the year still apply. At these times if the absence of carbohydrate snacks and the restricted amounts of carbohydrates at lunch and dinner are making it difficult for you to control your eating, then switch to the basic serotonin-seeker's diet from Chapter Five. You will still lose weight; it just won't happen as quickly. What is more important is that you will be in control of your eating. Once you bounce back to your spring-summer mental mode you can go back to this diet plan.

7. Exercise. If you have already started some muscle building and toning, continue it, increasing either the frequency of the workouts and/or the amount of the weights. Make sure that you check with a trainer first to prevent injuries.

Take advantage of every opportunity you have to move. Extended hours of sunlight make evening walks a pleasure. Long weekends provide time for recreational exercise. If you live in a climate that is so hot and humid that outdoor activity in the summer is absolutely foolhardy, there are other options—air-conditioned malls, health clubs, and tennis courts, for example.

How often should you exercise? Despite the continuing controversy about how much physical activity is needed for good health, it's pretty obvious that the more you move, the more muscle you will build and sustain. And that means the more calories you will burn. You have about six months to lose weight and get in shape before the days become appreciably shorter. By June 23 there are already a few minutes less of daylight than there were on June 20. There isn't any time to waste.

CLOUDY DAYS, CLOUDY MOODS

What do you do if there's a rainy spring and summer? There have been times when it rains or turns foggy and cold all spring. Then summer arrives and the days turn humid and hazy, with clear, dry, sunny days remaining at a premium.

When this happens you will still feel like a hibernating bear. Only now you feel worse than ever because your emotional immune system, worn down by winter, sorely needs an infusion of bright sunlight to renew both your spirit and your serotonin.

I had a colleague at MIT who was on sabbatical from a university in Jerusalem. All winter he complained about the miserable Boston weather. He was right: That winter was a particularly vicious one. We kept telling him that summer would be very warm; all he had to do was get through the winter.

The summer came. And, as promised, it was very warm. In fact, it was hot and humid and topped by a temperature inversion that turned the sky a sickening yellowish gray for weeks at a time. The poor man became extremely grumpy and blue. He kept saying that at home the summer days were reliably the same with blue skies, dry air, and cool nights. "I thought the winters here were bad," he told us. "But I would trade any winter day for the gloomy weather we're having now."

He started to exhibit all the signs of winter depression. Feeling lethargic, he lost interest in his work. Every afternoon he was seen heading to a nearby bakery for an infusion of chocolate chip cookies. The lack of bright sun due to the constant cloud cover and smog had the same effect on him as the short days of winter have on so many others. He had a mild case of SAD—in a different season.

Researchers who study SAD and the winter weight-gain disorder have records of patients who go through an entire year without a remission. Weather is usually to blame. If there is no sunlight because of bad weather conditions, it won't matter how many hours there are between sunrise and sunset. You will still feel as depressed as if it were the middle of January and the sun was setting at 4:15 P.M.

If you are living through one of these summers, then the spring-summer slim-down plan may be hard to follow. If that is the case use the serotonin-seeker's diet all the time. While it contains about two hundred or so calories more than the summer slim-down plan, it will still allow you to lose weight while providing the carbohydrate boost you will definitely be needing.

CHAPTER NINE

The Shift-Work Diet

Many of us do not work a standard nine-to-five schedule. In our society, which operates around the clock, as many as one in four people may work either an evening shift from 4 P.M. to midnight, a night shift from midnight to 8 A.M., or a second job that extends the work "day" well into the evening. Some of these people may also have to work different shifts from week to week.

Nearly every business has extended its hours. It's not just hospitals, police stations, firehouses, and airlines that require the services of shift workers; now almost all service and marketing companies offer twenty-four-hour access—and round-the-clock workers to provide it. If someone wants to open a bank account, send flowers, or order electronic equipment at 2 A.M., he can.

There are the people whose workday extends across several time zones. A financial manager I know in San Francisco awakes at 5 A.M. in order to deal with his counterparts in New York City. If he is planning to do business in Europe—nine time zones away—he has to get up even earlier.

There are many people whose jobs require extended work

Much of the information that appears in this chapter comes from the document titled "Prevalence and Use of Shift Work," published by the Office of Technology Assessment, Government Publication Office, Washington, D.C., 1991.

hours: lawyers preparing for a trial, accountants at tax time, politicians running for office, and so forth. And then there are the people who take night courses. A young woman I know who is attending law school at night understands this phenomenon all too well. When asked when she sleeps she replied, "In the summer."

We humans are biologically programmed to wake with the sun and sleep when the sun goes down. And, until artificial light became available, that is what we did. Ironically, even though we take for granted that just about anything we want or need will be available on a twenty-four-hour basis, our society still behaves as if everyone works during the day and sleeps at night. Traffic reports, heard frequently during rush hours, are scarce at 11 P.M. Apartment dwellers are told to keep their televisions and radios at a decent level after 10 P.M.; no one tells them to keep the noise down after 10 A.M. Prime-time hours on television are always in the evening, never during the night workers' early-afternoon leisure period. With rare exceptions, restaurants close before midnight in most cities and don't open again until 6 A.M. or later. Even hospitals and factories with twenty-four-hour shifts do not offer equal support facilities to their night workers. One complaint I heard frequently from nurses working the 11 P.M. to 7 A.M. shift at a local hospital concerned the absence of any place to buy nutritious food or get some fresh air and exercise (although this hospital does provide noon aerobics classes). There's not even a safe place to take a walk. The lovely grass quadrangle used by daytime personnel for lunch and breaks becomes a hangout for muggers and drug addicts at night. The hospital cafeteria closes at 10 P.M. By midnight even the vending machines are empty. So the nurses end up eating the candy and cookies brought in by friends and families of the patients, food that most of the patients don't feel well enough to eat themselves and so give to the nurses. "I don't know how many nights I have dined on fancy chocolates and tins of cookies," one nurse told me. "If I could convince the patients' families to bring big tossed salads and slices of lean roast beef I would really have something good to eat."

Working after-hours in an office building or a factory poses the same problems. Even if someone brings in take-out food, the choices in the middle of the night are limited and generally heavy on fat and calories, and low on nutrition.

STRESS AND THE INTERNAL CLOCK

Each day there are specific times when our body temperature rises or falls, periods when hormone secretion reaches a peak or drops, and moments when we become hungry or thirsty, sleepy or alert. These daily rhythms are regulated by our internal biological clock, which, it is believed, is set by the pineal gland, and keyed to the passage of light and darkness.

Anyone who has ever crossed time zones is well aware of these internal rhythms, because they make it so difficult to force our bodies into a new sleep-wake schedule. I remember a trip to France with my husband when I awoke in the middle of the night feeling frantically hungry. It was about 2 A.M. and room service had long since ceased. As I searched through my purse and carry-on bag, hoping to find some forgotten package of crackers, my husband awoke, also starved. Now the two of us were on a search and devour mission for food—any kind of food. Finally he found a snack in his briefcase. It was enough to satisfy our immediate hunger and we went back to sleep. The next morning, however, when it was time to eat breakfast we weren't hungry at all. The problem was that our internal rhythms were out of sync. Our appetites were still on U.S. Eastern Standard Time. We had awakened hungry the night before at what would have been our normal dinnertime. We weren't hungry in the morning because breakfast time in France coincided with the hours when we would have been asleep back home. It didn't matter what Paris time was; our bodies were running on their own internal schedules.

It is one thing to endure the slow transition the body will make to a new time zone when on vacation. It is quite another to have to endure this transition while working. People who must cross time zones often complain of not feeling well all the time. They are constantly tired, their stomachs are upset, and they suffer from perpetual headaches or muscle soreness. I know a man whose job required him to commute from Australia to Boston every six weeks. He told me that, after two years of travel, he suffered such severe burnout that he could not work for over six months and finally had to change jobs. "Forcing my body in and out of time zones was like forcing my foot into a shoe that was too small," he told me. "I found my memory deteriorating. I walked around with chronic headaches, feeling depressed and anxious. It took me months of living in one place and not traveling to feel like myself again."

It is not necessary to fly across the ocean to feel a disruption of your biological clock. Shift workers suffer similar problems. Their schedules can run like this: working 7 A.M. to 3 P.M., switching to a 3 P.M. to 11 P.M. shift, and then to an 11 P.M. to 7 A.M. shift (or vice versa). Studies, many sponsored by the federal government, report emotional and physical stress is extremely high among shift workers. Depression, tension, mental and physical fatigue, digestive problems, and overeating and weight gain are typical problems. Surveys of industrial accidents show that more occur between 2 and 4 A.M. than any other time. It is possible that the mental slowdown thought responsible for these occurrences is due to the difficulty of continuously adjusting to sleep-wake cycles totally out of sync with the body's internal rhythms.

SHIFT WORK AND WEIGHT GAIN

Weight gain is one of the shift worker's most common problems. The stress of feeling physically and mentally uncomfortable from having to adjust to a constantly changing shift provokes overeating as the brain's way of forcing the body to consume enough carbohydrates to boost the serotonin stress-relief system.

However, shift workers, as well as individuals whose work requires traveling to different time zones, gain weight because they try to use food as both a sleeping and a wake-up aid. And food can be quite effective at doing these jobs, but only if you eat the right kinds and amounts of food according to a precise schedule. Unfortunately, many people who use food as stimulants or sedatives don't understand this, and they end up gaining a lot of weight (and still not sleeping well or feeling alert during their waking hours).

One example of this dilemma is a woman who came to me for weight-loss counseling because she had put on seventy-five pounds during the previous year. A dispatcher for the transit police, she told me that she knew her weight gain was due to her extremely erratic, demanding work schedule. From week to week this woman never knew how many days she would be going to work at 9 A.M. or 11 P.M., or even how long her shift would last. Some weeks she worked eight hours at a time; others, she was asked to do a double shift of sixteen hours. There was never time to adjust. She said she couldn't remember what it felt like to be rested and energetic. Even her days off were exhausting as she raced to do her errands and keep all the appointments that had piled up. She ate to stay awake and ate to go to sleep. And she ate too much.

This is how she described a typical day. If she was on a night shift, she ate a muffin or a sandwich at home around 10 P.M. to wake herself up for the drive to work. Once there, she plugged herself into her computer lines; she could not leave the station unless another dispatcher covered for her. Access to food, however, was not her problem, since there were ample supplies readily available—pastries, doughnuts, soft drinks, coffee, and sometimes either carry-out pizza or Chinese food that someone had brought in. Because she started to feel sleepy around 3:30 or 4 A.M., she always ate a big meal then to try to wake herself up. (This is the time when the body really slows down and wants to rest.)

Around 6 A.M., she ate whatever her fellow workers on the

next shift had brought in, usually doughnuts, muffins, or bagels and cream cheese. Then, if she didn't have to work longer, she went home.

The idea of going to sleep right away seemed impossible, which is entirely normal. Few people who work night shifts can fall into bed as soon as they arrive home. Instead, in the morning she did her chores: cleaning, marketing, returning phone calls, and checking through the mail. Around 11 A.M. she made herself something to eat, like a sandwich and soup or eggs and toast, and then, finally, she went to sleep. When she awakened in the late afternoon she cooked dinner for herself and her husband, and they ate when he got home around 6 P.M. Then she had a snack with him about two hours later, lay down for a brief nap, woke up at ten, ate her sandwich or muffin, and went off to work.

When asked about exercise, her reply was a short "Never." She didn't have time and was chronically too tired to even think about it. Short staffing at work also meant she couldn't even take some time off just to walk around. That's why she ate her 3 A.M. snack at her desk.

Working against the clock does not have to cause overeating and weight gain, and it does not have to cause exhaustion either. By following the multifaceted plan I have developed, you will be able to reset your body's internal clock and minimize the bad effects of shift work or travel.

There are four ways to push the body into a sleep-wake cycle of your choice: food, sleep, sun and darkness, and exercise. My plan makes use of all four.

FOOD: THE-EATING-BY-THE-CLOCK PLAN

Eating certain kinds of food can make us feel more mentally alert and vigorous, while other foods help us unwind and relax. The eating-by-the-clock plan is a guide to selecting foods that work on the brain to promote wakefulness when you must be awake and drowsiness when you must sleep.

It is also a carefully designed weight-loss plan, since so many shift workers are overweight. However, it can also be used for weight maintenance, by simply adding four hundred to six hundred calories per day, including one or two additional food exchanges. Easy-to-use and completely flexible and adaptable, the food guide can be followed even if your eating timetable is constantly being disrupted because of changing shift schedules or travel. There is, however, one obstacle to the success of the food plan: You will have to force yourself to eat when your body would prefer to sleep, and vice versa. You *must* do so because your appetite mechanisms are on the standard night-day sleep-wake cycle. This internal schedule makes sure that you feel the need to eat at least every five to six hours during the day but switches off your hunger at night. Otherwise, you would not be able to wait up to twelve hours until breakfast. If you follow my plan, you will be able to trick your body into a new pattern.

Don't be dismayed if you find it difficult to eat the foods recommended on the plan during the first few days. When you awake from a sound sleep at 3 A.M., it will take some willpower to get yourself to eat. You are going to have to force your body to behave in new and—for a while—uncomfortable ways. But you will soon see the benefits. Foods *can* help you make successful transitions to new waking and sleeping patterns and *can* alleviate the stress of working against your natural biological rhythms. The eating-by-the-clock plan is based on what we know from our research about how protein and caffeine stimulate brain chemicals to increase mental alertness and how carbohydrates help us relax and unwind. By following this plan, you will feel less stressed and more in control of your eating.

This is an unconventional plan because your eating needs are so out of the ordinary. Rather than giving you traditional meal and snack plans—what do you call an 11 P.M. or 4 A.M. meal anyway?—I am dividing all the food into two categories: foods for alertness that are to be eaten during waking-working hours, and foods for relaxation that are to be eaten after work. The alertness and relaxation foods can be eaten as part of traditional meals, or, if you prefer, they can be divided into many smaller meals. This flexibility is especially useful because you may not have regular break times or free times that are long enough to allow you to consume a whole meal. As long as you do not exceed the amount of food on the plan, you can eat as frequently as you wish.

Whenever you eat any of the starch exchanges you must eat protein along with them. On days you are working an extended schedule, keep eating the alertness foods; this is especially important if sleepiness threatens to ruin your concentration. Start eating the relaxation foods at least an hour or so before going to bed. In fact, if you don't have to drive yourself home, you might think about eating a relaxation food for a snack shortly before you leave work. That way the relaxing effect can start to kick in while you're on the way home. By the time you arrive, you will be calm and ready for bed.

Note that since the eating time and meal sizes for a shift-work plan are necessarily more flexible than in the other diet plans, these exchange tables are set up differently. You decide when you need either alertness or relaxation foods, and how much of each to consume at any given time. As long as your totals for each kind of food fall within the overall guidelines, you will be able to maintain energy, strength, and alertness when you need them and also unwind and fall asleep when you need to.

Caution: Beware of your internal clock tricking you into eating large meals at the wrong time. Typically, you might feel very hungry at the end of your shift, which could fall at midnight or early morning. On the way home from work you may be tempted to stop for a large cheese pizza, Chinese food, or a big breakfast of eggs, home fries, sausage, buttered toast, and coffee. If you have such a meal, don't plan on going to sleep. Your internal mechanism is making you hungry because it expects you to be getting up and going to work; at the very least it expects a few more hours of being awake. By eating so much food, you will be speeding up your metabolism. Instead of feeling drowsy and ready to sleep you will be restless, unsettled, and wide-awake.

Alertness Food Exchanges

6 protein (48 grams)
4 starch (60 grams)
3 vegetable (15 grams)
1 fruit (15 grams)
2 fat (10 grams)
total calories: 965

Whenever you eat any of the starch exchange foods on the alertness food list, make sure that you also consume some protein along with them. As you read in Chapter Two, when you combine protein along with carbohydrates, the amino acids in the protein prevent trytophan from getting into the brain. This means, of course, that no serotonin will be made. If you want to stay awake it's important not to activate the manufacture of serotonin, which is relaxing. If it's bedtime, it can make you sleepy. So don't eat the starchy exchange foods without protein until you are ready to unwind and get your body ready for sleep.

The following menus are for night-shift workers who need to be awake and alert in the predawn hours. Remember: Both the meal and snack designations and the times at which I've suggested eating them are *only* suggestions. Eat your alertness foods whenever and in whatever combination suits you.

NIGHT-SHIFT WORKERS' ALERTNESS FOOD SAMPLE MENUS

Wake-up Meal (5:30 to 6 P.M. can be the same as family dinner)

3 ounces baked chicken
$^1/_2$ cup noodles

1 cup string beans
1 cup salad consisting of dark green leafy lettuce, 1 chopped
    carrot, 1 tomato, $^1/_2$ cucumber
$^2/_3$ cup tomato juice
Equals: 3 protein, 1 starch, 3 vegetable

or

omelet (two egg whites plus one whole egg, red peppers, and
    onions, cooked in nonstick pan)
1 slice low-fat cheese
1 turkey sausage
2 slices tomato
1 slice whole wheat toast
1 orange
Equals: 3 protein, 1 starch, 1 vegetable, 1 fruit

Before-Work Snack (9 to 9:30 P.M.)

1 cup fat-free fruit-flavored yogurt
$^1/_2$ cup low-fat granola
1 cup coffee (with fat-free milk if desired)
Equals: 1 protein, 1 starch

or

1 slice bread
1 ounce turkey luncheon meat
1 tablespoon fat-free mayonnaise
half tomato
lettuce
Equals: 1 protein, 1 starch, 1 vegetable

Mid-Point Work Meal (2 to 3 A.M.)

1 cup vegetable soup (take in thermos or add boiling water to
    dehydrated soup)

2 ounces chicken or turkey
6 rice minicakes, white cheddar flavor
1 carrot
$^1/_2$ sweet red pepper
1 cup coffee, optional (with fat-free milk if desired)
Equals: 2 protein, 2 starch, 1 vegetable

or

1 low-fat frozen lunch*, if microwave is available (check label
    for grams of protein and carbohydrate)
1 apple
1 cup coffee, optional (with fat-free milk if desired)
Equals: 2 protein, 2 starch, 1 fruit

or

1 container microwaveable beef stew* or chili*, if microwave
    is available (check label for grams of protein and
    carbohydrate)
2 large rice cakes
1 carrot
$^1/_2$ zucchini, cut into sticks
1 pear
1 cup coffee, optional (with fat-free milk if desired)
Equals: 2 protein, 2 starch, 1$^1/_2$ vegetable, 1 fruit

After 2 to 3 A.M. you will choose selections from the relaxation
foods. It will take about an hour or so before you will feel their
relaxing effect, so eat them soon before you are about to end your
work shift.

*Read package labels to make sure foods inside meet the exchange
  requirements.

Relaxation Food Exchanges

5 starch (75 grams)
1 fruit (15 grams)
1 fat (5 grams)
total calories: 505

NIGHT-SHIFT WORKERS' RELAXATION FOODS SAMPLE MENUS

Last Snack Before Work Ends (6 A.M.)

$^1/_2$ cup orange juice
2 large caramel-coated, or any other flavor, rice
    cakes
Equals: 2 starch, 1 fruit

or

1 cup instant hot chocolate (made with water)
3 fat-free sugar cookies
Equals: 2 starch

Back Home Meal (8 A.M.)

$1^1/_2$ cups hot oatmeal
1 tablespoon maple syrup
1 4-ounce glass orange juice
Equals: 3 starch, 1 fruit, 1 "free"

or

2 slices whole wheat toast
1 teaspoon peanut butter
1 tablespoon jelly

1 orange
Equals: 3 starch, 1 fruit, 1 fat, 1 "free"

or

2 toaster waffles
1 tablespoon syrup
$^1/_2$ banana, sliced
Equals: 3 starch, 1 fruit, 1 "free"

or

$1^1/_2$ cups sweet breakfast cereal like Cinnamon Toast Crunch
$^3/_4$ cup blueberries (keep frozen until ready to eat)
1 cup herbal or decaffeinated tea or decaffeinated coffee
Equals: 3 starch, 1 fruit

EVENING-SHIFT WORKERS' ALERTNESS FOOD SAMPLE MENUS

Late-Morning Meal (10 to 11 A.M.)

1 toasted waffle
$^1/_2$ cup cottage cheese
1 cup strawberries
1 cup coffee (with fat-free milk if desired)
Equals: 1 protein, 1 starch, 1 fruit

or

1 three-inch pita
1 slice fat-free ham
1 slice low-fat cheese
1 orange
1 cup coffee (with fat-free milk if desired)
Equals: 2 protein, 1 starch, 1 fruit

or

2 ounces water-packed tuna mixed with celery, pickles, and
     fat-free mayonnaise
$^1/_2$ sliced tomato
$^1/_2$ sliced cucumber
$^1/_2$ sliced sweet red pepper
2 slices whole wheat bread
1 cup low-fat or fat-free milk
Equals: 3 protein, 2 starch, 1 vegetable

At-Work Meal (5 to 6 P.M.)

If you have prepared food for your family, bring a portion for
yourself. Or, if you don't like preparing a regular meal for
one, buy cooked foods. There's a wide variety available from
supermarket deli counters and salad bars. Frozen or dried microwaveable meals are another option.

3 ounces sliced chicken
1 cup dehydrated lentil/rice soup
1 container of cut up raw vegetables, such as sweet red pep-
     per, carrot sticks, red cabbage
1 banana (small)
coffee, tea, or diet soda
Equals: 3 protein, 2 starch, 1 vegetable, 1 fruit

or

crabmeat salad sandwich roll (4 ounces of mock crabmeat,
     1 tablespoon fat-free mayonnaise, 1 chopped carrot,
     $^1/_2$ thinly sliced red pepper, lettuce, half of a 6-inch
     pita)
1 orange
Equals: 4 protein, 2 starch, 1 vegetable, 1 fruit

EVENING-SHIFT WORKERS' RELAXATION FOOD SAMPLE MENUS

Snack (10 P.M.)

1 cup instant hot chocolate (made with water)
1 ounce package fat-free pretzels
Equals: 2 starch

or

1 snack pack of Fig Newtons
1 cup of herbal tea
Equals: 2 starch

or

1 cup decaffeinated coffee (with fat-free milk if desired) or
decaffeinated tea
5 fat-free biscotti (18 calories each)
Equals: 2 starch

Before-Bed Meal

$^3/_4$ cup blueberries
2 toaster waffles
1 tablespoon blueberry-flavored pancake syrup
Equals: 2 starch, 1 fruit, 1 "free"

or

2 slices whole grain bread
1 small banana, sliced
2 teaspoons peanut butter
Equals: 2 starch, 1 fruit, 2 fat

or

2 blueberry or apple-filled frozen blintzes cooked with
    nonstick spray
1 cup melon chunks or 1 chopped apple sprinkled with
    cinnamon
Equals: 2 starch, 1 fruit

or

1 baked sweet potato
$1/4$ cup chopped dried apricots
decaffeinated tea with 1 teaspoon sugar
Equals: 2 starch, 1 fruit

The alertness and relaxation food menus can be adapted for use by people traveling through time zones. To accelerate your adjustment to a new time zone, you should eat the foods on the alertness food list until evening, and then switch to the relaxation foods for dinner—no matter how hard it is to eat when you want to be sleeping or to eat breakfast foods when you long for a substantial dinner.

RECIPES

Alertness Omelette

1 egg
2 egg whites
$1/4$ cup red bell pepper, chopped
3 scallions, chopped, including green tops

Whisk together egg and egg whites and pour into a medium-sized nonstick sauté pan. Cook over medium heat until the surface just begins to bubble and the edges to cook. Add the pepper and scallions. Fold the omelette in thirds, turn, and cook two more minutes.

"Breakfast" Burritos

For a delicious change of pace:

Serves 4

> 1 carton egg substitute
> 1/4 teaspoon prepared mustard
> fresh ground pepper to taste
> 3/4 cup any combination chopped onions, tomatoes, and peppers
> 4 slices low-fat cheese
> 4 6-inch flour tortillas, at room temperature

Spray a nonstick skillet with a small amount of vegetable spray. Add the egg substitute, spices, and vegetables, and cook over medium heat as you would scrambled eggs, stirring frequently to prevent sticking, about four minutes. Divide the mixture equally over the tortillas, top with a piece of cheese, and roll up. Wrap each tortilla in a paper towel and microwave on high for thirty seconds. Serve with lots of hot sauce.

Super Sandwich

This sandwich can be made ahead and eaten either cold or warmed up in a toaster oven. Eminently portable, it can also be sliced and eaten in portions to suit your appetite.

> 1 medium-size Italian or French roll
> 2 slices fat-free ham
> 2 slices fat-free cheese
> 1/2 cup mixed vegetables, such as sliced mushrooms, onions, peppers, and tomatoes; season with sprinkle of oregano
> 1 teaspoon olive oil

Layer the roll with slices of ham and cheese. Sauté the vegetables in 1 teaspoon olive oil until tender. Top the sandwich with the vegetable mixture.

Relaxation Fries

These spicy "unfried" fries are a real treat after a long shift.

1 large baking potato, washed but not peeled
light vegetable oil cooking spray
1 large egg white
2 tablespoons Cajun spice mix

Preheat the oven to 400 degrees. Slice potato into ¼ inch slices, then slice lengthwise into thin matchsticks. Coat a nonstick baking sheet with three sprays of vegetable spray. Combine the lightly beaten egg white with the spice mix. Toss with the potato sticks to coat evenly and well. Spread in a single layer over the baking sheet and bake on the bottom rack of the oven for forty to forty-five minutes, turning often with a spatula as the potatoes begin to brown and get crisp. Serve immediately.

Late-Night Linguini

Serves 2

12 ounces pasta
1 10-ounce box frozen chopped spinach
3 cloves garlic, minced
2 teaspoons olive oil
¼ cup chopped fresh basil, or 1 tablespoon dried
fresh ground pepper
1 to 2 tablespoons low-fat Parmesan cheese

Cook the pasta according to package directions. Meanwhile, cook the spinach according to package directions or microwave. Add the garlic, oil, and basil to the spinach and continue to heat two more minutes. When the pasta is done, drain and toss with the spinach mixture. Top with freshly ground pepper and cheese. Serve yourself 2 cups of pasta mixture.

AVOIDING TROUBLE

1. Take the time to think about what you are going to eat, both at home and at work. Give yourself adequate time, either on days off or at home, to prepare and pack the food you will be eating at work. Bring food from home or stop at the supermarket on the way to work.

2. Do your food shopping on days off when you have some time to make a list of the meals you will be taking with you to work. Make sure you have appropriate containers, including insulated lunch boxes and frozen coolants to keep foods from spoiling.

3. Keep some food staples at work in case you get so busy at home that you don't have time to prepare anything. Flip-top cans of water-packed tuna, containers of dehydrated soups, chili, stews, macaroni and beef, even high-protein sports bars are all good emergency rations to keep in your locker, desk, or office refrigerator. Add a few bags of rice cakes or pretzels, small containers of yogurt, milk, and juice, a few apples or bananas, and instant coffee—all of which can usually be bought at twenty-four-hour convenience stores. You will have enough food to last through several meals. (A can opener, a small electric teapot that boils water if your workplace does not have a hot water dispenser or microwave, plastic utensils, and disposable bowls are also useful to have on hand.)

4. Buy food from an all-night supermarket if you were unable to prepare meals in advance and your emergency stash is gone. The salad bar may or may not be set up in the middle of the

night, but there will still be plenty of good foods from which to choose. The deli counter has cooked food; fruit, vegetables, dairy products, and healthy drinks are all available. It doesn't take much longer to get a turkey sandwich made at the deli counter than to wait for a pizza to be warmed up at a take-out place. Buy vegetables and fruit and small containers of yogurt. Not only will the meal cost less than the pizza: You will be better nourished and much more alert.

5. Pay attention to what you eat when leaving work. It can be very difficult for you to wind down enough so that you can go to sleep soon after arriving home. Food and darkness help; going out with your coworkers for a big breakfast does not. Isn't it more relaxing to be home, munching on some soothing carbohydrates in a darkened room with soft music playing, rather than crammed in a noisy restaurant filled with diners about to go to work? The energy level, conversation, and food are all geared to workers about to begin their work-days. You, on the other hand, are more than ready for a day's rest. Go home.

SLEEP: THE SEROTONIN CONNECTION

You must get enough sleep and it must be uninterrupted rest, not a series of naps. But many shift workers deprive themselves of sleep, because they need to use the daylight hours to take care of personal, social, family, and practical obligations. With so many of the services we depend on obtainable only during the day, sleep may be the first thing to be sacrificed.

Unfortunately, lack of sleep is a powerful overeating trig-ger. When you attempt to resist the need for sleep, your brain may signal a demand for carbohydrate foods. But these carbohy-drate cravings are not only caused by the needs of your stress-management system. Your brain is issuing a call for serotonin because it is a key element in another brain system, the one that puts us to sleep. If you try to resist the brain's signal for sleep and stay up, you may begin to feel an intense hunger for carbohydrate foods. If you eat carbohydrates when your internal clock wants you to sleep, the food will act like a sleeping pill.

Recently I was speaking with a physician colleague who said his constant traveling was causing him to gain weight. When I asked why, he replied that he was constantly sleepy from jet lag. He never stayed in one place long enough to adapt to a new time zone. "I find myself eating carbohydrates all the time," he told me. "Bread, rolls, pastries, candy—something is always going into my mouth." Then I asked him if these foods woke him up. "No," he answered. "I am constantly sleepy and I eat to try to keep myself going." He was shocked when I told him that his carbohydrate hunger was his body's way of pushing him into sleep. But then he agreed that this was exactly what was happening.

Insufficient sleep isn't the only reason you feel exhausted and hungry for carbohydrates. Lack of sleep will also affect mood. Anyone who is sleep deprived, or whose sleep is broken in the middle of the normal sleep cycle, will agree. I once lived in an apartment building whose fire alarm system malfunctioned, always in the middle of the night. For months the residents were awakened at 3 or 4 A.M. by a loud, obnoxious, recorded voice telling us a fire alarm had gone off and to stay in our apartments. This message would be followed by ten minutes of beeps, horns, and bells. Then the voice would come on again. Then the sounds. After thirty minutes of this we learned it was a false alarm.

The morning after you risked your life if you ventured a "good day" to another resident. People do not appreciate interrupted sleep—and they show it.

Depression, anxiety, and tension due to broken or shortened sleep simply intensify the urge to overeat, especially carbohydrates. Your brain will be seeking serotonin for the dual purposes of relieving stress *and* getting you to sleep. *Remember: Sleeping too little means eating too much.* Allow yourself to get the rest you need. It is one of the most important things you can do to control your eating.

SUN AND DARKNESS

The rhythms of the human body respond naturally to the twenty-four-hour cycle of day and night.

Currently there is a considerable amount of ongoing research to see whether light and darkness can be used to speed up adjustments to new work schedules. Although strategies designed to readjust the internal clock so that it will operate on a different pattern from the one it is accustomed to are only partly effective, this is what is known. Complete darkness during daylight hours helps the body adjust to sleeping in the daytime. And, conversely, bright artificial lights have been shown to make people feel more alert, perform better, and experience a greater sense of well-being when they have to be awake at night. Studies carried out with astronauts aboard the space shuttle *Columbia* found that bright-light treatment helped the night-shift crew feel less exhausted and better able to concentrate.

If you need to sleep during the day, eyeshades and special room-darkening blinds will produce almost total darkness. Remember also to cover any digital clocks, VCRs, or other devices with lighted surfaces. This is extremely important since any light can trigger your awakening responses. Once you are awake, you might consider using a phototherapy unit to fool your body into thinking it is sunrise. Phototherapy devices supply controlled amounts of bright light that imitate the early morning light of spring and summer. Often prescribed as therapy for people who suffer from the mood changes of seasonal affective disorder and winter weight gain (see Chapter Eight), phototherapy light boxes are widely available and may range in price from around $250 to $500, which may even be covered by your health plan. Information about suppliers of light boxes and their use in shifting sleep-wake cycles can be obtained from:

Society of Light Treatment
10200 West 44th Avenue, Suite 304
Wheat Ridge, CO 80033-2840
Phone: 303-424-3697

Part of our information on whether light therapy can shift our body's rhythms comes from research on volunteers who were exposed to light or darkness for varying lengths of time to see how their internal body clocks were affected. Shift workers agreed to try exposure to phototheraphy boxes at different times to see how much light was needed to shift their daily rhythms. Early results seem promising, but as yet, no large-scale trials have been undertaken.

Someone who has to be awake during nighttime hours should sit in front of the light box soon after awakening, for at least thirty minutes and up to an hour if possible. Since some of these boxes simulate dawn, they might be particularly useful in fooling the body into thinking that the sun is rising, even at night.

In the spring and summer, a low-tech solution to the problem of adjusting to nighttime work hours is to go outside in the afternoon or early evening and expose yourself to natural light before going to your job. In the fall or winter, it will be dark when you awake from your daytime sleep. Using a phototherapy unit during those months may help.

EXERCISE

Exercise increases your rate of metabolism and can fool your body into feeling more awake. When your temperature, heart, and breathing rates go up, your body edges closer to the way it would normally feel during the day. Many business travelers who cross time zones use exercise as a quick way of waking up their bodies—and, they hope, their minds—especially when the new business day is beginning at what feels to them like 1 or 2 A.M.

The exercise should be aerobic. A casual stroll or stretching will not affect breathing, heart rate, or body temperature sufficiently to make much difference to an internal clock. The duration of the exercise doesn't matter as much as speeding up the metabolism. So working up a sweat—or at least feeling warmer than you did when you began—is important. In an ideal night-shift workplace you would have access to a gym during the 3 A.M.

break in order to renew physical and mental vigor with a short round of strenuous exercise.

If you have an exercise bicycle or treadmill at home, dust it off and use it. You can do two to four bouts of exercise, five to ten minutes each, in between chores. Exercising with a video or audio tape will also speed up your metabolism, as long as it features more than stretching and limbering. Going to a health club or the Y will not only give you more variety in your exercise routines but also will help energize and motivate you by exposing you to music, lights, and the activities of lots of other sweaty bodies.

The increased mental and physical vigor you feel after exercising will help you get into your new sleep-wake schedule more quickly. The exhaustion, irritability, and stress you tend to feel during the adjustment period will decrease. So, too, will your need to consume carbohydrates to subdue your discomforts. You'll be eating fewer calories, burning more of them thanks to the exercise, and losing weight.

FACING UP TO STRESS

It is very tempting to use alcohol as a quick way of relaxing after you come home from a shift. Indeed, it is not unusual for people to have a few beers at seven in the morning as a way of unwinding. The hazards of such drinking go far beyond its caloric impact of one hundred calories per ounce of alcohol. Don't use alcohol to get yourself to sleep after your shift is over. Even though small amounts, like a glass of wine, will make you feel relaxed and sleepy, too much alcohol disrupts normal sleep patterns. When you awake you will feel even less rested than usual.

Two jobs, one job plus school, or one never-ending job all are sources of stress that extend beyond lack of sleep and time; your body and brain are being forced to perform for too many hours without any down time to rest and recover. The inevitable weight gain in cases like these can't be fixed by eating protein at 3 A.M. or sleeping with an eyeshade.

All of us go through periods in which work takes over our lives and there is nothing we can do about it. If the excessive demand on our time has a beginning and end, we can usually endure it. We know that our routine will eventually return to normal. But if the demands seem to be without end, then so is the stress, along with the potential for overeating and weight gain. Fixing a problem of this magnitude may require more serious solutions, like changing jobs or getting help with your after-work obligations. The proverb "You cannot burn the candle at both ends" really applies to the shift worker.

CHAPTER TEN

The Ex-Smoker's Stress Plan

Cigarettes and eating: Stop one and start the other. For millions of people who have quit smoking—or very much want to—weight gain is a major fear. With good reason: Eating excessive quantities of food, especially carbohydrates, is almost a given among ex-smokers in the first two or three months after quitting. Weight gain is so common that its absence is considered abnormal.

Statistics on weight gain confirm what the ex-smoker already knows from experience: The average former smoker puts on about five to seven pounds. However, as many as twenty or more pounds may be gained during the initial three- to six-month period. A study published in the *New England Journal of Medicine* in November 1995 went even further. After surveying nearly six thousand people, the study reported that people who had quit smoking within the last ten years were significantly more likely to become overweight and stay that way compared to those who never smoked. The results also showed that 16 percent of the men and 21 percent of the women who had quit smoking within the past ten years gained thirty-three pounds or more. Although the study did not examine why ex-smokers were more apt to gain weight than those who never smoked, the reason may be simple.

Every time they were upset, irritated, annoyed, or angry, ex-smokers may have replaced smoking with snacking. And a chain smoker who turns into a chain eater can put on a lot of weight.

Ex-smokers know that, without their cigarettes, they are doubly likely to gain weight. The stress of giving up cigarettes will cause them to eat more. But, just as important, they have given up nicotine, a powerful drug that suppresses appetite. Any smoker who has lit a cigarette instead of having dessert, or even a meal, knows how effectively nicotine dampens hunger. It is no wonder that people who have used cigarettes to keep their weight low or to help them lose weight are so fearful of the consequences of giving up nicotine.

While no one knows how many ex-smokers return to cigarettes because they have gained weight, my suspicion is that the number is extremely high. And certainly the fear of gaining weight is intense, as I learned from studies that Dr. Bonnie Spring and I carried out at MIT over the past few years. Like many other researchers, we wanted to find effective ways to minimize weight gain among ex-smokers. About four years ago, we began a study to see whether the experimental drug dexfenfluramine might relieve the hunger pangs of the ex-smoker.

After we placed a newspaper advertisement stating that we were trying an experimental medication to prevent weight gain among those who had just quit smoking, we were inundated with phone calls. To our dismay, many of the callers decided not to join the study because we couldn't guarantee that they would receive the drug. We were doing a double-blind study, in which half the volunteers would be given a placebo and the other half would get the drug. No one—neither the volunteers nor the staff who administered the study—would know who was in which group until the end. (That's the meaning of "double blind.") When we told them there was a fifty-fifty chance they might receive a placebo, many were no longer interested. "I can't risk gaining any weight," one woman told us. "I don't care how dangerous it is to smoke. I would rather be thin."

Others lost interest when we informed them that it wasn't

known for certain whether the drug would prevent weight gain. We explained that while the drug was likely to do so, since it had been shown to decrease the tendency to overeat, no one had ever tested the drug on those who had just quit smoking. Even this degree of uncertainty was too much. A number of women therefore declined to join the study, saying that even a one- or two-pound gain was unacceptable.

Then there were the women who managed to stay off cigarettes throughout the three-month study, despite the extremely unpleasant symptoms of nicotine withdrawal. Although they admitted they felt wonderful once the nicotine was out of their bodies, a number of them told us they were going to start smoking again. These women had gained an average of five or six pounds; they knew diet and exercise would remove them fairly easily, but, as one volunteer explained, "It's easier to smoke. That way losing weight will be less of a hassle."

STRESS AND THE EX-SMOKER

The stress of giving up cigarettes accounts for most of the weight gained by the ex-smoker, but it is a special kind of stress, caused by nicotine withdrawal. The effects of nicotine withdrawal on mood cannot be overstated. Because nicotine is a drug with potent effects on the brain, specifically on the serotonin stress-management system, when a person quits smoking he or she is bound to go through considerable physical turmoil. Ex-smoker stress probably ranks higher than all the other stresses described in this book. It can last for weeks—if not months. The ex-smoker is emotionally fragile and frequently has difficulty concentrating, remembering, sleeping, and exercising emotional control. Although the intensity of emotional distress varies from individual to individual, some people experience a constant state of distress lasting throughout the withdrawal period—and beyond. Some ex-smokers claim that their nicotine craving never ceases. They wake up in the middle of the night yearning for a cigarette months after they have stopped smoking. Many told me that when a major catastrophe, such as serious illness, divorce, death, or severe financial problems occurred, it was almost impossible for them not to resume smoking. And many did begin again.

For people who use cigarettes to prevent themselves from responding to unpleasant emotional situations, giving up cigarettes can be brutal. One subject in our study was doing extremely well; she was not smoking and had gained very little weight until five weeks after she had quit. Then she put on three pounds in one week and started to smoke again. Why? She had had to attend the annual reunion of her husband's family.

As she related to me after the event, she detested all the family members and the feeling was returned in kind. In the past she had been able to control herself by smoking, rather than fighting. "Every time I wanted to say something nasty I would smoke. I think I went through two packs in one afternoon. But at least I kept my mouth shut."

But this year was different. With no cigarettes to stick in her mouth, she ate instead. Whenever she wanted to answer an insult she would eat. But by the end of the afternoon she was so full that she could not get anything else into her stomach. She gave in and started to smoke.

She acknowledged that her inability to communicate anger was a real problem, one which she had been able to camouflage when she smoked. And she decided after talking to me that she was going to seek psychotherapy to work out this problem, because she did not want to solve it by permanently going back to cigarettes.

CIGARETTES NO; WEIGHT GAIN YES

The relentless need to eat, brought on by the stress of nicotine withdrawal, accounts for most of the weight put on by ex-smokers. But weight is gained for other reasons, too. Nicotine has a well-established effect on metabolism. Researchers who measure changes in metabolic rate before and after smoking cessation agree: Nicotine increases metabolism; withdrawal of the drug slows metabolism down. This means that when you give up cigarettes you burn fewer calories. However, your metabolism does not slow down to that of a two-hundred-year-old tortoise. It decreases by a mere one hundred calories a day—the equivalent of a medium-sized banana. When you stop smoking, if you do not change what you eat or how much you exercise, those one hundred calories should account for a weight gain of about ten pounds over twelve months, or less than one pound a month. Unless you put nicotine back into your system, you will not go back to the slightly higher metabolic rate experienced while smoking. But compensating for those extra one hundred calories is easy. Eliminating one banana, two rice cakes, or one slice of bread with a teaspoon of jam will take care of that amount. Exercising the calories off is even better. Ten minutes of moderate activity daily is all that's required.

At this point you are probably asking yourself—and me— then why does weight build so quickly? Why do I gain six or seven pounds a month every time I stop smoking? If my slower metabolism accounts for such a tiny weight gain, where did all those other extra pounds come from? The answer is simple. The pounds pile on because the ex-smoker is eating too much.

As someone who had never smoked, I had no firsthand experience of how rapidly the ex-smoker turns into a perpetual eating machine. But when our subjects came in for their weekly visits and behavior-modification sessions, I observed how obsessively they ate. They looked like they were on a video that was playing in fast-forward mode.

The most vivid example that I saw of their prodigious food intake occurred during the group meetings held in our offices. We provided a large variety of low-fat or fat-free foods. The conference table was covered with bowl after bowl of popcorn, pretzels, licorice sticks, gumdrops, Gummi Bears, fruit chews, and fat-free cookies. We put out much more food than we thought necessary. But it was never enough. Women who had been thin when they smoked, who never used to overeat, were now inhaling these snacks. By the end of a ninety-minute meeting the only thing left uneaten were a few kernels of unpopped corn.

The former smoker spends a lot of time eating or thinking about eating, because eating is an activity that keeps the hands and mouth very busy. The ritual of smoking requires a considerable amount of hand-to-mouth action. Just watch someone open a pack of cigarettes, light one up, tap the ashes between inhalations, and move the cigarette continuously back and forth—gesturing with it, putting it down, picking it up again, and so forth. After quitting smoking what can the ex-smoker do to occupy his or her hand and mouth? Eating meets this requirement wonderfully well.

Another reason for overeating is that eating breaks replace smoking breaks. Smokers use cigarettes as a means of giving themselves a brief respite from work. This is especially true these days when you have to leave your desk or workstation and go to a special room or even walk outside the building to smoke. For someone accustomed to having a cigarette as a reward upon the completion of a task or as a way of interrupting a tedious job, giving up this built-in "recess" is difficult. Having a cup of coffee and a few cookies in the break room or wandering down to the vending machine for a candy bar may be a poor substitute for a social interlude with your fellow smokers, but at least it gets you away from work for a few minutes.

One of our study volunteers told me she found it extremely hard to complete her self-imposed chores at home after she gave up cigarettes. "When I smoked, I motivated myself to do something tedious, like ironing, with the promise of a reward when I was finished. So now I reward myself by sitting down, having a cup of tea, and eating a few pieces of toast while I look through a magazine. If I know I have that to look forward to, I can motivate myself to keep working."

This woman defined the classic behavior pattern of the former smoker. If you can't use smoking to take a break from your activities, then you will use eating as a convenient substitute. It's easy to see how quickly one can gain weight if instead of tea and toast you eat a candy bar or a bag of chips every time you want a cigarette. Turning from a pack-a-day smoker to a several-bag-a-day chip eater will slowly but surely add to your increasing girth.

THE SEROTONIN CONNECTION

The specifics of the mechanism by which smoking cessation and nicotine withdrawal affect mood and appetite have to do with—you guessed—serotonin. Nicotine is able to act on the same cells that normally respond to serotonin. However, nicotine is so much more powerful than serotonin that during the smoking years the smoker's cells almost stop responding to serotonin, learning to rely instead on nicotine to run the stress-management system. So whenever the smoker feels the need to decrease stress, improve mood, or become more focused or relaxed, the usual response is to light up.

And it works because nicotine communicates very effectively with many of the chemical messengers (neurotransmitters) the brain uses to maintain optimal function.

If the smoker stops smoking, the brain cells no longer have access to the nicotine they depended on to maintain emotional well-being. Although serotonin is, of course, available, the smoker's brain cells have been desensitized to it by the years of exposure to nicotine and can no longer respond to serotonin.

The entire stress-management system begins to fall apart and the ex-smoker feels it, badly, in the form of insomnia, irritability, restlessness, difficulty in concentrating, spaciness, anger, and depression. All these and more are typically reported, especially during the first two or three weeks after quitting.

Appetite is affected as well. The only way the brain can make the cells respond to serotonin is to flood them with very large quantities of it. The brain is now desperately seeking tryptophan to make a lot of serotonin. You have a voracious appetite for sweet and starchy food on top of the emotional turbulence caused by a dysfunctional serotonin stress-management system and—just to make things really unpleasant—an intense longing for cigarettes. That's stress.

THE CARBOHYDRATE-CONNECTION STUDIES

The excessive appetite for sweet and starchy carbohydrates in ex-smokers has been recognized for many years. One of the first researchers to point it out, Dr. Neil Grunberg of the Uniformed Services University of the Health Sciences (the military's medical school in Bethesda, Maryland), interpreted it as the ex-smokers' response to the stress of not being able to smoke. Only recently has this eating pattern been linked to the brain's need for serotonin.

In one of the earliest attempts to confirm this link, researcher Dr. Bonnie Spring did a double-blind study in which she gave part of a group of ex-smokers a placebo, and the other part a dose of tryptophan. The ex-smokers who were treated with tryptophan reported significantly better moods than did those who were given the placebo.

Dr. Spring and I then collaborated on a series of studies with women who were going through the various stages of smoking withdrawal to see how their food choices, weight, and moods changed immediately after they gave up cigarettes and then again after several weeks of being abstinent. We also were interested in whether their increased appetite and weight gain could be minimized by the use of dexfenfluramine.

As expected, appetite and food consumption increased dramatically in the days and weeks after quitting smoking. However, three months later we could see a real difference between the group that was getting a placebo and the one taking dexfenfluramine. While still consuming more sweet and starchy foods than they had before quitting smoking, those on the drug ate much less food, especially sweet and starchy snacks, than those in the placebo group. They also gained fewer pounds. It appeared that the drug was able to help the brain recover from the devastation caused by lack of nicotine. We could not know exactly what was happening inside the brain, but we speculated that perhaps the drug was restoring the serotonin stress-management system to its pre-nicotine levels. The brain no longer had to make larger than normal amounts of serotonin to compensate for its ineffectiveness after nicotine withdrawal. And because the need for extra serotonin was reduced, the ex-smokers lost their "carbohydrate thirst."

We could tell that dexfenfluramine was affecting the serotonin stress-management system in another way as well. Many of those receiving the drug had tried unsuccessfully to give up smoking in the past, and they told us that this time it was much easier for them. They kept waiting for the familiar symptoms to begin, wondering when their good moods would vanish, to be replaced by the anger, irritation, impatience, and lack of concentration they had experienced before. But it never happened. Some told us that, if they had known how easy it was to quit, they would have done it long ago.

One subject had a particularly dramatic response to the drug treatment. A highly respected professional, she was extremely hardworking, impatient, and somewhat abrasive. Telling us at the beginning that she was entering our study under duress, she said she really didn't want to stop smoking. It turned out that her coworkers were pressuring her to quit because her smoking was disrupting the flow of work. Since she was not allowed to smoke in her office, she had to walk quite a distance to get outside to have a cigarette. These interruptions were a constant source of friction between her and her coworkers who relied on her presence in the office. We were concerned that the hardship of going through smoking withdrawal would make it even more difficult for her to get her work done. Her complaints about participating in our study made us assume that she would withdraw at the earliest opportunity.

We were wrong. Within a matter of days her entire perspective and personality changed. She felt wonderful, always smiling, never missing a session. More important, she never smoked. Her eating habits changed very little and whatever weight she put on was insignificant. Her only "complaint" was that she felt so relaxed that she stopped feeling guilty for time taken away from work.

Interestingly, I bumped into her at an airport about two years after the study. She recognized me and, after saying hello, told me that she hadn't touched a cigarette since the study began. She said she had gained between seven and ten pounds and was planning to exercise to lose them.

Not surprisingly, at the study's end it had turned out that she was one of the ones who had been taking the drug. The ease with which she gave up cigarettes and her ability to resist overeating were almost certainly due to dexfenfluramine's serotonin-enhancing effects. Those who hadn't taken it but had been on the placebo experienced the full range of unpleasant effects that are part of nicotine withdrawal.

We now feel that the serotonin-deadening effects of nicotine withdrawal are behind the whole cluster of mood and appetite changes experienced by the former smoker. In the period after nicotine leaves the system and before serotonin returns to normal, the urge to overeat carbohydrates is so strong that even serotonin-boosting drugs like dexfenfluramine can't entirely control it. Since the drug cannot manufacture serotonin, but can only enhance the activity of what is already there, the ex-smoker is still left with the need to eat carbohydrates.

THE NICOTINE PATCH

In the early nineties several drug companies began to market nicotine patches. Placed on the skin, the patches delivered a constant dose of nicotine over a twenty-four-hour period. The patches came in series that contained three different amounts of nicotine, in graduated doses. The ex-smoker started with the highest-dose patch and, over three or four months, moved to the intermediate and finally to the lowest dose. When coupled with an educational program to support the user in withdrawing from cigarettes, the nicotine patch was very effective. Unfortunately, many people did not take advantage of these programs. Also, some of the programs did not continue over the full three months of patch usage. In those cases, the ex-smoker who still had weeks to get through often became discouraged, tossed the patch, and picked up a pack of cigarettes.

Curiously, nicotine patches had no effect on preventing an ex-smoker's increases in appetite and tendency to gain weight, although they did help alleviate the actual cravings for nicotine. This doesn't mean that the patch shouldn't be tried. When used correctly, with educational support, it can be extremely helpful. But it does mean that the former smoker must still contend with the problem of weight gain.

NICOTINE WITHDRAWAL AND WEIGHT GAIN: DEALING WITH THE INEVITABLE

Although miracles do happen, it is unlikely that anyone going through a nicotine-withdrawal period is going to lose weight or even be able to maintain an existing weight. I wish it were otherwise. Nothing would please me more than to be able to tell you that, by following the ex-smoker's-stress food plan, you won't gain weight. I can't—because for most people it won't be true. The enormity of the stress and the severity of the serotonin disturbances that occur during the first five or six weeks after quitting smoking mean it is almost psychologically impossible for you to summon the willpower to refrain from overeating. Your brain, devastated by nicotine withdrawal, is unable to use the full power of your stress-management system. Without it, no self-discipline, no matter how intense, can overcome the urgent need for serotonin. And no willpower is going to quiet the incessant demand by the brain that you consume large amounts of carbohydrates to repair the damage inflicted by nicotine.

You will be eating more than you were while smoking. And you will weigh more, too. But—and this is the good news—if you follow my ex-smoker's-stress food plan, that weight gain should not be more than five pounds—and probably even less.

I realize that, to many of you, even a few unwanted pounds

are unacceptable, even though you know they will vanish once your eating is under control and you exercise regularly. I can hear you saying, "I would rather risk my health than walk around with fat hips and a bulging stomach."

Whenever I encounter someone who is unwilling to gain a few pounds in the short run to make a long-term improvement in health I always think of a famous routine of the late comedian Jack Benny, whose stage persona was that of a man who never willingly parted from his money. A thief snarled to Benny, "Your money or your life," only to be met by a very long silence. When the robber repeated his threat with even greater urgency, Benny finally responded, "I'm thinking, I'm thinking."

Funny or not, the person who is making the crucial decision to smoke or not to smoke has to make the same kind of decision. Perhaps this will help to reassure you: Although weight gain may indeed be unavoidable, the ex-smoker's-stress food plan makes it possible to keep weight gain to an absolute minimum during the first two or three months after quitting. At that point you should begin to feel comfortable as a nonsmoker. Your stress level should be returning to normal, your brain no longer demanding that carbohydrates be eaten around the clock. Now will be the time to lose the weight you gained, and you can go on the weight-loss plan in Chapter Five, which will help you to lose it easily.

Probably every lapsed smoker has a story about how some intolerably stressful event caused him or her to light up again. *The Serotonin Solution* gives you the means to prevent this from happening. The food plans have been created to reduce stress and the overeating that stress inevitably generates. If, in the future, you find yourself in a crisis situation, dying to have a cigarette, use food, rather than nicotine, to supply the calmness, comfort, and relief you are seeking.

THE EX-SMOKER'S-STRESS FOOD PLAN

Simplicity was the goal of this plan, and simple is what it is. It will provide you with frequent doses of low-fat or fat-free carbohydrate food so that your brain stops desperately seeking serotonin. That means you will not be craving a cigarette to make yourself feel better. Also, the plan requires very little willpower on your part; giving up cigarettes is enough of a struggle. At about 1,900 to 2,000 calories, the plan is designed to minimize weight gain, rather than achieve weight loss. Save the dieting for later.

My approach is this: You have to eat—all the time. In order to keep any weight gain to a manageable minimum I have made sure portions are not too large, and fat and calorie contents are low. Just as in the past you always had to have a pack of cigarettes with you, now food will be your constant companion. Wherever you go, a carbohydrate snack should accompany you. This is especially important because it's not as socially acceptable to bum a bagel as it is to bum a cigarette. If you are not eating, then you should be engaging in other cigarette-substituting behaviors. These include sipping water or dietetic beverages like iced tea or soda, or chewing on something nonedible, like a coffee stirrer or gum.

If you wake up in the middle of the night wanting a cigarette, you should eat. Be prepared. Keep a package of crackers or a single-serving-size box of dry cereal next to your bed along with a small thermos of cold water or decaffeinated iced tea. Your body must realign its systems to function without a drug you have been supplying it with. This takes time, and the readjustment will continue even when you are asleep. Feelings of depression, agitation, anger, or even loss can hit strongly during the night. You can, however, eat your way through them. By keeping a snack-sized "dose" of carbohydrates with you at all times, you will be able to respond immediately to the call for more serotonin. And by planning those snack selections ahead of time, you'll be able to make sure that your "doses" are chosen from among the low-fat low-calorie items on the grocery shelves.

Smoking puts extra nutritional demands on the body, such as an increased need for vitamins like C and E and for minerals, including calcium. Until your body becomes accustomed to the absence of nicotine, its need for these nutrients may remain high, which is why this plan calls for particularly nutrient-dense foods. If you are unable to eat the variety of foods that will naturally supply these nutrients, make sure you take a daily vitamin-mineral supplement. Also pay attention to your food choices; don't waste calories on selections that are geared only to your taste buds. The sample menus provided will give you some ideas of the types of food to eat.

The ex-smoker's-stress food plan should begin on the day you quit and can be continued for as long as you feel it is needed. It is hard to predict just how long it will take your body to readjust. Even if you have stopped smoking in the past, your reactions may differ this time.

The first two weeks are the toughest, making the most demands on your eating control. Your body is convalescing, restoring itself, and it will take a while before you begin to feel better. As your body adjusts to the absence of nicotine, the need to eat excessive quantities of carbohydrates will gradually lessen. Eventually you will regain control over both your eating and your mood. At that point you can stop the ex-smoker's-stress food plan and switch to the serotonin-seeker's diet (see Chapter Five).

I have been asked by more than a few smokers why they can't diet at the same time they give up cigarettes. Their attitude was perfectly understandable. Since the pain of giving up nicotine was so great, they thought they wouldn't even notice the ache of food deprivation. Unfortunately, it doesn't work that way. The battering that nicotine withdrawal inflicts on the serotonin stress-management system is too overwhelming. You can't simultaneously deprive yourself of cigarettes *and* of sweet and starchy carbohydrates. If you don't eat enough carbohydrates to meet your brain's demands, how can your stress-management system be restored? Without carbohydrates your mood changes will be so ugly that not only will your friends and family want to avoid you, you won't want to have anything to do with yourself either. And your cravings for both carbohydrates and cigarettes will continue to haunt your life.

One more time: Your top priority should be to stop smoking. Once that is accomplished, with a minimum of weight gain, weight loss can begin.

Drink as much water as you can. Nicotine withdrawal may make you thirsty, so sip water continually throughout the day and keep a carafe or thermos by your bed at night. Your daily liquid intake should be at least ten eight-ounce glasses.

Many smoking-withdrawal programs recommend that their members do not drink coffee because it's associated, for many people, with their first cigarette of the day. If you think by not drinking coffee you will more easily break the morning smoking habit, then by all means, avoid it. However, if avoiding coffee—and the caffeine it contains—causes its own withdrawal symptoms, such as headaches, then don't add to your physical woes. Find another way of shunning that early morning smoke.

SAMPLE MENUS

Breakfast Exchanges

1 protein (8 grams)
2 starch (30 grams)
1 fruit (15 grams)
total calories: 290

Breakfast

1 cup dry cereal (a mixture of high-fiber bran and other
     types)
1 cup low-fat or fat-free milk
$^1/_2$ grapefruit
coffee or tea as wanted
Equals: 1 protein, 2 starch, 1 fruit

or

1 fat-free bran muffin
2 teaspoons apple butter (a thick applesauce-like spread, con-
    taining no fat)
$^2/_3$ cup cranberry juice
1 cup fat-free, sugar-free yogurt
coffee or tea as wanted
Equals: 1 protein, 2 starch, 1 fruit

Mid-Morning Snack

a sweet or starchy food containing 40 to 45 grams of carbo-
    hydrates and no more than 210 calories.

Mid-Morning Snack

2 cups of apple-cinnamon Cheerios, $1^1/_2$ cups Cinnamon
    Toast Crunch cereal, *or* 18 apple-cinnamon flavored rice
    minicakes

Lunch Exchanges

2 protein (16 grams)
2 starch (30 grams)
3 vegetable (15 grams)
1 fat (5 grams)
total calories: 420

Lunch

chef's salad (1 ounce turkey chunks, 1 ounce fat-free cheese
    strips, 1 red pepper in strips, 1 sliced cucumber, 1 cup
    spinach leaves, 1 shredded carrot, $^1/_4$ cup drained chick-
    peas [starch exchange], $^1/_4$ cup drained kidney beans

[starch exchange], 4 black olives, 1 cup shredded red cabbage, 2 tablespoons fat-free dressing)
Equals: 2 protein, 2 starch, 3 vegetable, 1 fat

or

1 3-inch pita roll-up sandwich (1 ounce cooked chicken, 1 ounce fat-free cheese, $1^1/_2$ cups mixture of broccoli, onions, mushrooms, and red pepper, sautéed in 1 teaspoon olive oil. Broil or microwave until cheese is melted.)
Equals: 2 protein, 2 starch, 3 vegetable, 1 fat

or

1 cup vegetable soup
1 ounce mock crabmeat salad with fat-free mayonnaise
3-ounce bagel, toasted
1 cup cabbage slaw (shredded cabbage and carrots with fat-free dressing)
1 cup fat-free sugar-reduced yogurt
Equals: 2 protein, 2 starch, 3 vegetable

Afternoon Snack

same as mid-morning snack

or

2.5-ounce package red licorice sticks and one Tootsie Pop

or

10 Bit-O-Honey candies (individually wrapped, not the candy bar)

or

5 Nips (long-lasting hard candies in assorted flavors like coffee, chocolate, and peanut butter)

or

any gummie candies that are the equivalent of forty to forty-five grams of carbohydrates

or

saltwater taffy: read labels to calculate how much to eat

Dinner Exchanges

2 protein (16 grams)
3 starch (45 grams)
2 vegetable (10 grams)
1 fruit (15 grams)
1 fat (5 grams)
total calories: 535

Dinner

1 cup spaghetti and meat sauce (recipe on page 211)
$1/2$ cup steamed spinach with garlic olive oil (recipe on page 211)
$1/2$ cup grated carrot salad with fat-free dressing
1 baked apple
Equals: 2 protein, 2 starch, 2 vegetable, 1 fat, 1 fruit

or

2-ounce swordfish kabobs with red and green pepper, onions, mushrooms, and tomatoes (recipe on page 212)

2 small ears of corn
steamed string beans
$^1/_2$ cantaloupe
Equals: 2 protein, 2 starch, 2 vegetable, 1 fruit, 1 fat

or

2 ounces of stir-fried lean beef with onion, garlic, 1 red
    pepper, 1 carrot, $^1/_2$ cup mushrooms, and tomato sauce
    atop small 3-inch pizza crust
tossed salad
1 pear
1 teaspoon olive oil
Equals: 2 protein, 2 starch, 2 vegetable, 1 fruit, 1 fat

Evening Snack

same as mid-morning snack

If you haven't had enough dairy products during the day,
have an 8-ounce glass of low-fat or fat-free milk.

The evenings will be particularly troublesome for many, since that
was the time for smoking while you relaxed, watching television
or reading. Without cigarettes to occupy your hands and mouth,
you will feel the need to nibble almost constantly. Pick sweet or
starchy snacks that take a long time to eat. Examples are: air-
popped fat-free popcorn, a Sugar Daddy (a caramel lollipop), fat-
free granola, miniature marshmallows, chocolate or fruit-flavored
sprinkles (eat them with your fingers), licorice whips, Charleston
Chews, Necco wafers, frozen fruit juice bars, frozen fudge pops,
fat-free biscotti or rusks, frozen orange segments dipped in fat-free
chocolate sauce, and frozen blueberries.

If you awaken during the middle of the night craving a cigarette and can't get back to sleep, try drinking a cup of herbal tea
with one tablespoon of sugar. If you feel the need to eat, have any

sweet or starchy fat-free carbohydrate that is handy; you'll want to get back to sleep as quickly as possible.

RECIPES

Chef's Salad

This is so big and attractive, you probably won't be able to eat it all at once.

Serves 1

2 ounces turkey
1 slice fat-free cheese
1 red pepper, cut into strips
1 cucumber, sliced
1 cup spinach leaves, rinsed
1 carrot, shredded
1/4 cup chickpeas, drained
1/4 cup kidney beans, drained
1 cup red cabbage, shredded
2 tablespoons fat-free salad dressing

Toss ingredients together in a large salad bowl and serve.

Stuffed Pita Sandwich

Serves 1

2 ounces cooked chicken
1 slice fat-free cheese
1 cup cooked broccoli
1 scallion, chopped, including green top
1/2 cup cooked mushrooms

1 pimiento pepper, sliced
1 6-inch pocket pita

Combine the sandwich ingredients. Halve the pita and stuff with the filling mixture. Broil for two to three minutes or microwave on high for forty-five seconds, or until cheese is melted and sandwich is heated through.

Steamed Spinach with Garlic Olive Oil

Serves 2

Do use fresh spinach for this recipe when in season. It makes all the difference.

2 cups fresh spinach, rinsed and lightly shredded
or
1 10-ounce package frozen spinach, thawed and pressed to remove excess moisture
2 cloves garlic, crushed
1 tablespoon olive oil
salt and pepper to taste

Place the spinach leaves in a medium saucepan with 2 tablespoons water. Cover and cook over low heat until wilted. Add the crushed garlic to the hot spinach and toss to distribute evenly. Drizzle with olive oil and toss again. Season to taste with salt and pepper.

Spaghetti and Meat Sauce

Don't be afraid to try a simple Italian jar sauce for this, but be sure to check the label for added starch or sugar.

Serves 2 to 3

6 to 8 ounces uncooked spaghetti
light vegetable oil cooking spray
1/4 pound lean hamburger
1/2 cup onion, chopped
3 cloves garlic, crushed
1/2 cup mushrooms, sliced
2 cups Italian-style tomato sauce
1 teaspoon oregano
1/2 teaspoon marjoram
1/2 teaspoon rosemary
salt and pepper to taste

Prepare spaghetti according to package directions. While it is cooking, lightly coat a nonstick skillet with vegetable spray. Add the lean hamburger and continue cooking until lightly browned. Add the onions and garlic and continue cooking until the onions are transparent. Add the mushrooms and tomato sauce, along with the remaining seasonings. Simmer twenty minutes. Drain the pasta and spoon sauce liberally over to serve.

Swordfish Kabobs

Lightly marinated in nonfat dressing, these grilled wonders are a treat all year long.

Makes 2 kabobs

4 ounces swordfish cut into 1-inch chunks
1 red pepper, seeded and cut into 1-inch chunks
1 green pepper, seeded and cut into 1-inch chunks
1 red sweet salad onion cut into chunks
6 fresh mushrooms, cleaned
2 tablespoons nonfat balsamic vinaigrette (see page 161)
1 teaspoon sesame seed oil

Combine the above ingredients in a large bowl. Toss with vinai-grette and allow to marinate at least one hour. Thread chunks on skewers and grill or barbecue ten minutes on each side.

Baked Apples

Sweet and so satisfying. . . .

Serves 4

4 large firm apples, cored (Granny Smith)
6 tablespoons dark brown sugar
1 teaspoon cinnamon
$1/2$ teaspoon nutmeg
$1/4$ cup lite nondairy whipped topping

Preheat the oven to 350° F. Combine the sugar and spices, and fill the cored apples with the mixture. Bake uncovered for thirty to forty-five minutes. Allow to cool slightly, and serve with a dollop of whipped topping.

AVOIDING TROUBLE

1. Brush your teeth as frequently as possible. Anyone who eats a lot of candy should do this anyway.
2. Be aware of how much you are eating. Your patience isn't high enough to count strands of spaghetti or licorice, but that doesn't mean you should be eating with your eyes closed, figura-tively speaking. If you open a sixty-four-ounce bag of fat-free potato chips and demolish it, you should realize you ate too much. The same goes for cleaning out a gallon of fat-free ice cream or a box of fat-free breakfast cereal. Try to minimize your overeating. Read labels. Keep a calculator handy to figure out how many pieces or sticks or cups you can eat within your calorie

allocation. And notice serving sizes on labels. If the calories per serving seem suspiciously low, that's sometimes because the serving size is ludicrously small.

3. Learn to distinguish between eating to settle and soothe your mood and eating to keep your fingers and mouth busy. I call the latter "gnawing," an activity that should be satisfied with nonfood items. If, after you have eaten the prescribed dose of carbohydrates, you feel you must still put things in your mouth, then go for a nonfood. If you don't, and eat more, you most certainly will gain weight. A lot of choices are at hand: plastic or wood drink stirrers, ice cubes, plastic mouthpieces for cigarettes (without the cigarette, of course), unlit pipes, gum (especially bubble), and straws. Try the water bottle used by bikers, runners, and other athletes. Its drinking tube is hard enough to be chewed and if you drink from it frequently, you will be giving your body the water it needs. The bottles can be found in any store that sells sporting equipment.

4. Be sure to exercise. The restlessness and difficulty you feel in settling down, caused by nicotine withdrawal, can be worked out of the body through vigorous physical activity. If you find yourself pacing, tapping your fingers, or feeling on pins and needles, then go for a brisk walk, hop on a stationary bike, or, if your knees can take it, jump rope for a minute or two.

There are other compelling reasons to exercise. Strength training increases muscle mass, which means that when you begin your weight-loss regimen, you will lose pounds more quickly. This is why men lose weight faster than women—after puberty they have more muscle. If you rarely exercised while you were a smoker, your muscle mass may be very small. If you have never done any workouts with weights or machines that strengthen muscle, be sure to get some guidance from a professional trainer before you start. Once you know how to work your muscles you will be amazed at how quickly they will begin to develop.

Exercise will use up some of the calories consumed as you go through the early stages of smoking withdrawal. Take advantage of your newly smoke-free body and slowly begin to explore the types of strenuous exercise that were impossible in the past.

During the very early stages of smoking withdrawal you may not sleep very well. If you find yourself constantly fatigued it will be hard for you to feel motivated to exercise. Do it anyway. You will not feel any more tired after exercise than before; odds are that you will feel invigorated instead.

5. Take a vitamin-mineral supplement daily. Although the highly nutritious foods on this eating plan should meet your nutrient needs, there will be times when your mood or lack of time and opportunity will make it hard for you to eat correctly. A supplement will compensate for any lapse in your food choices.

6. Eat lots of bran or high-fiber vegetables as part of your usual diet, or take a fiber supplement. They come in liquid, pill, or wafer form. Nicotine affects the chemicals that regulate the motility of the intestinal tract. Once you stop smoking you may find that constipation is a problem.

7. Avoid the temptation to overeat in social situations by keeping your hands occupied. Hold a glass of carbonated water, chew on toothpicks or plastic stirrers, or grab a handful of carrot and celery sticks if you're lucky enough to find them available. Otherwise your hands might seek out an endless supply of high-fat high-calorie food.

8. Try new ways to define the end of a meal. If you always ended a meal with a cigarette, you used it as a signal to stop eating. Without it you may continue to eat until all the food is gone. The temptation may be especially dangerous if you used to smoke while you cleaned up after a meal, because you may now find yourself eating leftovers as well.

Instead, when you have eaten all you should, drink a glass of carbonated water or diet soda. That action can become the signal that a meal is finished. Or chew gum or suck on a lollipop or a piece of hard candy. If you like, crunch on some ice cubes. Whatever you do, make it a new habit to replace your old one.

A LAST WORD

One of the best things you can do for yourself is to take advantage of smoking-withdrawal behavior-modification groups during the acute phase of giving up cigarettes. Since some of these programs may not be long enough to deal with all the problems that arise during the second or third month after you stop smoking, try to find a support group to help you through this time as well. There are "smokers anonymous" groups that are run like Alcoholics Anonymous; in fact your local AA may know of them.

Smoking and drinking alcohol go hand in hand. Relearning how to drink socially without a cigarette is hard. Your hand may be drawn to the bowl of peanuts or chips. Often, you start smoking again. Do yourself a big favor and don't put yourself in this situation until your new nonsmoking status feels comfortable and your eating is under control.

CHAPTER ELEVEN

The After-Diet Eating Plan

After a diet, do you sometimes look wistfully at the new clothes hanging in the closet and wonder if the store will take them back? Do you find yourself loading up on junk food after each weigh-in at your weight-loss program? Do you feel as if there are two people inside you: one with tremendous motivation and willpower who diets and is willing to put up with deprivation, the other waiting at the starting gate to race to all the food once again?

If you answered yes to any of the above, then you can enroll in one of the country's biggest clubs: the post-diet bingeing club. All you have to do to gain membership is binge after your diet is over. Many people who went to weight-loss programs belong; indeed, practically everyone who has ever been on a diet can claim membership.

Two things usually happen at the end of a diet: You pack up the food scale and exercise bicycle, and you open up the junk food vault. How soon before this happens varies. For some, the period can be painfully short. We surveyed obese volunteers applying for a weight-loss study to learn how rapidly they had started to regain their weight after their last diet. The majority answered that within two weeks they found themselves overeating again, and the foods they sought out were classic high-fat snack items like chips, cookies, ice cream, candy, and French fries. It turned out that whether or not they lost control after the diet was over was not related to the type of plan they had been on. Some had been on very restrictive regimens; others on more permissive, higher-calorie programs.

Although half of them had participated in maintenance programs, the ones who took the maintenance courses did no better than those who hadn't gotten any instruction. Eating control seemed to vanish when they felt stressed, angry, depressed, tense, irritable, restless, or profoundly out of sorts.

Regardless of the type of diet they had followed—and all current varieties were present—they felt defenseless against their urges to binge on excessive amounts of fatty, carbohydrate-rich foods soon after their weight-loss programs had ended.

THE SEROTONIN CONNECTION

Most high-protein low-fat low-carbohydrate diets leave ex-dieters totally vulnerable to weight gain. None of these diets provide sufficient carbohydrates to boost serotonin. Even diets that offer carbohydrates at meals rarely allow the dieter to eat substantial amounts of sweet or starchy foods by themselves. Between-meal snacks of sweet or starchy carbohydrates, even the low-fat ones I recommend, are even more uncommon. I have yet to see a commercial diet plan that recommends eating an ounce and a half of candy corn or eight candy pumpkins as an afternoon snack. Nor have I encountered one that recommends that you satisfy your need for an evening snack with an English muffin and jam or a few fig cookies and a cup of hot chocolate.

All of this means one thing: Your serotonin stress-management system becomes weaker as your diet proceeds, making your brain increasingly vulnerable to stress and increasingly insistent in its demand that you eat large quantities of sweet and starchy foods.

In our survey, the dieters who had been on low-calorie-formulated diet drink programs seemed to regain their weight most quickly. This may have been because the diet drinks were very high in protein and contained relatively few carbohydrates. Every time these dieters ate, their bloodstreams were flooded with the amino acids that prevent tryptophan from getting into the brain.

Sadly, all the dieters had a similar interpretation of their after-diet weight gains. All assumed that their inability to obey the laws of healthy food choices and portion control meant that they lacked self-discipline and willpower. A few had almost gotten to the point where they had given up on trying to lose their excess pounds, deciding that perhaps they were destined to be fat (this was prior to the discovery of the gene theory of obesity) and it was akin to tampering with fate to attempt to lose weight over and over again. A few wrote on the survey questionnaire that they believed their overeating was caused by their bodies trying to get back to their original set points. (Of course they probably didn't consider that their true set points were their long-ago pre-obesity weights.)

All were angry at themselves and bitterly disappointed at the failure of yet another diet program. What none of them realized was that their overeating had little, if anything, to do with person-ality, psychological history, set points, or defense mechanisms. It was almost entirely caused by the loss of their brain's power to halt food intake especially when they were emotionally distressed. And of course they couldn't know that their negative feelings were also caused by a weakening of their mood-regulatory system.

In other words, they had eaten themselves into a serotonin deficit.

A particularly poignant example of the inability to brake a binge was related to me by a young woman who asked to see me for a consultation in the middle of an after-diet binge. She had been on a low-calorie liquid diet for about five months and was within fifteen pounds of her goal weight when she started on the binge. Never before had she been able to lose so many pounds so quickly. Now in her late thirties, she was very happy. She had fi-nally found something that worked. And she knew her diets: She had been on and off dozens since her late teens.

But a month before her liquid regimen was scheduled to end, just before she was scheduled to start a refeeding program that featured regular foods, something had gone terribly wrong. She couldn't stick to the liquid diet any longer. Instead, she felt compelled to eat boxes of cookies and bags of corn chips, among other things. All her self-control was gone. She felt she was being driven, against her will, to eat the very foods she knew would ruin her diet. That was the point at which she called me.

When she gave me a typical day's rundown of just what she had been consuming, I was amazed. It was hard to believe that she could eat as much as she did, especially after surviving on a mere 450 calories a day for five months. In addition to consuming the four daily diet drinks (which she was afraid to stop because they symbolized the road back to self-control), she ate two jelly doughnuts, a large bagel with cream cheese, an order of lo mein, an Italian sub, a large frozen yogurt cone, and a bag of chocolate-chip cookies. To wash it down she drank several cans of diet soda. That took her to about 7 P.M.

Then she went to the supermarket to purchase supplies to get her through the evening. While shopping she scarfed down almost a whole bag of potato chips and a large candy bar. She still managed to buy a box each of brownies and muffins, along with a frozen cheesecake. By the time she got home the chips were gone and she finally felt full.

She left the rest of the food in the car with the rationale that if it was outside the house she wouldn't go near it. Then she fell asleep. At 1 A.M. she was up, looking for more food. The middle of the night found her sitting in her car, eating the groceries she'd left there.

When I asked her to describe her feelings during the binge she used the words *agitated*, *depressed*, and *angry*, and said that it seemed as if her body had been inhabited by another entity. The week preceding the binge she had been extremely irritable, was having trouble sleeping, and felt depressed even though the diet had been going well. All that week she'd found it impossible to erase thoughts of food from her mind.

"I knew I was going to lose control," she confessed. "That's why I had to see you. I feel as if my mind has been messed up. Even at my heaviest I never felt such a powerful urge to eat the way I'm eating now. It's like I'm in the eye of a storm, totally helpless, completely powerless against this force. Something bad has happened to my mind and mood. In fact, I'm seriously considering going to see a psychiatrist; I think I'm suffering from a chemical imbalance."

Ironically, she *had* diagnosed herself: She was indeed being tormented by a chemical imbalance. However, unlike imbalances associated with mental illness and of unknown origin, this one could be traced: The culprit was her diet plan.

THE RESEARCH

The brain is exquisitely sensitive to what we do or don't eat. Some scientists are now using this information to explain changes in behavior they see after weight loss; others are using the data to bring about mood changes experimentally by manipulating diet itself.

A few years ago a group of researchers in Edinburgh, Scotland, led by Professor Philip Cowan, published a study in which they made indirect measurements of serotonin activity in the brain before and after a three-week weight-loss program. The men and women who participated in the study were put on a 1,200-calorie-a-day regimen. Their carbohydrates were not severely restricted but were limited to fruits and vegetables.

The scientists then measured blood levels of the hormone prolactin, whose synthesis is regulated in part by brain serotonin. Changes in prolactin levels in the blood are a way of assessing alterations in brain serotonin. Also, they monitored the moods of their subjects throughout the study. In their published account, they stated that the subjects become steadily more depressed throughout the weight-loss program—even though they were losing weight—and that measurements of prolactin indicated a decrease in serotonin activity. The authors concluded that because of its meager carbohydrate content, even a diet that was not extremely low in calories could quickly lead to serotonin depletion. This could easily result in a depressed and agitated state. Of course, the same lack of serotonin would also lead to a fragile eating-control system. The inability to control eating on top of a diet-induced depression made for a volatile combination. An explosive binge was the inevitable result.

Confirmation of the effects of carbohydrate-restricted food plans on mood *changes* has come from another source as well. A Canadian researcher, Professor Simon Young, has been carrying out experiments for years in which volunteers are asked to follow a diet specifically designed to deplete brain serotonin. They consume drinks made of amino acids that are missing the one amino acid needed for serotonin production—tryptophan. After a day on a tryptophan-free diet, the volunteers report feeling depressed, agitated, restless, anxious, and stressed. Their serotonin stress-management system seems to have been rendered completely inactive.

Why hasn't such information been used to develop weight-loss plans that are serotonin protective? This data is so new that it has circulated only among psychiatrists, brain scientists, and psychologists, and is just now beginning to trickle down to those who are involved with eating disorders. Several researchers, including Dr. David Jimerson in Boston and Dr. Walter Kaye in Pittsburgh, are actively studying the role of serotonin depletion in provoking bulimia. They, like other scientists, believe there is a close connection between lack of serotonin and the depressed mood and impulsive eating that characterize this eating disorder.

WHAT DOES ALL THIS MEAN TO YOU?

First and foremost, none of the diet plans in this book deplete serotonin—they all increase it. When following any of them you don't have to worry about feeling depressed, angry, or stressed. But the after-diet eating plan is a particularly potent serotonin producer, designed to counter the effects of weeks or months of serotonin deficiency. So if you are now ending a conventional carbohydrate-restricted diet and are beginning to wonder "Now what do I do? Am I going to binge when I stop?"—this plan should put your mind at rest.

Maybe you have had to go on a severely limited diet because medical concerns necessitated a rapid weight loss. For example, you might have had an orthopedic problem, relief of which depended on how quickly you could shed pounds. Now that the weight is off you don't want to binge your way back to pre-diet levels. And you don't have to. What you must do is follow the after-diet food plan for a week to ten days after stopping your diet. It is a weight-maintenance plan containing about 1,800 calories a day. (The number will be lower if you use a purified protein powder as your protein food for breakfast and lunch.) The plan will take you from a state of carbohydrate and serotonin deficiency to one of sufficiency. You will neither gain nor lose weight. Please note, however, that if your diet was extremely low in carbohydrates, you *will* be replacing the water weight you lost within the first week or so of starting the diet. This will amount to about five to seven pounds—but it's water, not fat. So don't be alarmed. Although the scale may show a higher number, it doesn't mean you are any fatter, just as you weren't any thinner when you initially lost the water weight.

THE AFTER-DIET FOOD PLAN

This plan has one major goal: to restore serotonin levels to normal as quickly and effectively as possible. The diet should be used for seven to ten days. By that time you should be feeling a return of eating control and a lessening of diet-induced tension, irritability, and restlessness.

The therapeutic basis for the diet plan is this: Each meal contains sufficient quantities of carbohydrates to elevate the tryptophan in the blood and bring it into the brain where it will be used to manufacture serotonin. Moreover, the meals are carefully timed to ensure a long-enough interval between protein and carbohydrate consumption so that the protein can't slow down the serotonin production.

Breakfast and lunch are each divided into two mini-meals. First you eat the carbohydrate portion, then you eat the protein portion an hour and a half later. Dinner contains very little protein relative to the amount of carbohydrate. For those of you coming off a weight-loss plan where the main course always featured four to six ounces of protein, it may seem that you are substituting one form of deprivation for another. Remember this meal plan has one objective only: to boost serotonin levels so that your resistance to bingeing will be strengthened. And keep in mind that you only have to bear it for a week or so.

If you eat an early dinner, then eat the carbohydrate snack about an hour before going to bed. For example, if you eat dinner at six, eat your snack between 9:30 and 10:30 P.M. Otherwise, eat a carbohydrate snack about 3 hours after lunch.

The fruits and vegetables can be eaten with either or both parts of breakfast and lunch and, naturally, dinner. This is true for the other components of the meal, too: fat, condiments, spices or imitation foods, and any beverages like coffee, tea, and non-caloric drinks.

The breakfast and lunch proteins should consist mainly of low-fat carbohydrate-free foods like fresh fish or fish canned in water (tuna and salmon), chicken, shellfish, fat-free cottage cheese, or hard-boiled egg whites.

If, however, it's logistically difficult for you to prepare a serving of protein mid-morning and mid-afternoon, don't give up; the easiest—and lowest-calorie—way of consuming protein is in a supplement drink. Sold in powdered form and marketed as protein supplements for athletes (and bodybuilders in particular), these are readily available in health food stores as well as many supermarkets and drugstores. There are several varieties that contain no carbohydrate or fat, are remarkably low in calories, and taste good. These include: ProMax, MLO Milk & Egg Protein, Pro Score 100, Diet Fuel, Max Muscl, and MLO Superhigh Protein.

(Avoid the dietetic meal replacement drinks like SlimFast and Sweet Success. Although they contain protein, they also have carbohydrates.) Read the labels carefully: Since you must limit your intake to about twenty-five grams (about the equivalent of one three-ounce can of tuna), and most of these products define a serving as fifty grams, you'll have to remember to cut the serving size in half when you're mixing it up—half the powder and half the liquid. If you like, you can blend the powder with fruit juice or fruit and count this toward your fruit exchange. Powdered coffee, flavor concentrates (extracts like vanilla, butter rum, chocolate, coconut, and almond), instant sugar-free hot chocolate mix (note calories and count them), and diet sodas mix well with the protein powder and make very palatable drinks. When you're going to consume these drinks at work, mix them ahead of time at home and carry them to the office in an insulated container. This is the least messy way of getting a well-blended drink. If you prefer to mix it at work, get yourself a tiny, battery-powered handheld mixer.

It is very important to separate the two parts of breakfast and lunch by ninety minutes to ensure that the mainly carbohydrate content of part one is digested before you eat more protein. Although it probably won't take an entire hour and a half to do this, I want to make absolutely sure that nothing interferes.

Do not go for more than four hours without eating carbohydrate. This is especially important to remember on weekends or vacation days when your schedule is apt to be less carefully structured.

In the sample schedule that follows, the recommended eating times are only suggestions. You'll vary the times to suit your own needs. But don't vary the *amount* of time between parts one and two of breakfast and lunch, and *do* eat either a late afternoon *or* an after-dinner snack.

	Weekday	*Weekend*
Breakfast: part one	7 A.M.	9 A.M.
part two	8:30 A.M.	10:30 A.M.

		Weekday	*Weekend*
Lunch:	part one	noon	2 P.M.
	part two	1:30 P.M.	3:30 P.M.
Afternoon snack		4:30 to 5 P.M.	
Dinner		6 to 7 P.M.	7:30 to 8 P.M.
Evening snack			10:30 P.M.

Part 1 Breakfast Exchanges

$^1/_2$ protein (under 4 grams)
2 starch (30 grams)
1 fruit
total calories: 255

Sample Part 1 Breakfast Menus

1$^1/_3$ cups hot oatmeal
$^1/_2$ sliced banana
Equals: 2 starch, 1 fruit

or

2 blueberry blintzes
$^3/_4$ cup fresh blueberries
Equals: 2 starch, 1 fruit

or

2 pancakes
1 tablespoon syrup
1 sliced orange
Equals: 2 starch, 1 fruit, 1 "free"

or

1 fat-free bran muffin
1 teaspoon fat-free cream cheese

1 sliced pear
Equals: 2 starch, 1 fruit

or

1 small toasted bagel
1 teaspoon jam
$^1/_2$ grapefruit
Equals: 2 starch, 1 fruit, 1 "free"

Part 2 Breakfast Exchanges

3 protein
1 fruit (15 grams)
total calories: 270

Sample Part 2 Breakfast Menus

1 glass protein shake containing 25 grams protein. Blend with
one fruit or mix with 6 ounces fruit juice
Equals: 1 protein, 1 fruit

or

1 cup fat-free cottage cheese
$^1/_2$ cantaloupe
Equals: 2 protein, 1 fruit

or

1 cup fat-free sugar-reduced yogurt mixed with $^3/_4$ cup fat-free
pineapple cottage cheese
Equals: $2^1/_2$ protein, $^1/_2$ fruit

Part One Lunch Exchanges

$1/2$ protein (under 4 grams)
3 starch (45 grams)
2 vegetable (10 grams)
total calories: 325

Sample Part 1 Lunch Menus

1 large baked potato topped with salsa
2 cups mixed salad, consisting of lettuce, tomato, carrot, and
    raw broccoli
1 tablespoon fat-free salad dressing
Equals: 3 starch, 2 vegetable, 1 "free"

or

$1^1/2$ cups cold rice or bulgur salad with 1 cup of chopped
    vegetables and fat-free dressing
1 cup tomato or vegetable soup
Equals: 3 starch, 2 vegetable

or

1 cup fresh sliced strawberries, blueberries, orange segments
    in $1/2$ cantaloupe
1 fat-free blueberry muffin
This menu substitutes fruit for the vegetable
Equals: 2 starch, 2 fruit

or

1 large bagel with 3 slices of tomato, alfalfa sprouts, 1 thin
    slice of red onion, fat-free mayonnaise
2 cups vegetable soup
Equals: 2 starch, 2 vegetable

or

1 large pita roll-up filled with stir-fried vegetables
1 small tangerine
Equals: 2 starch, 1 vegetable, 1 fruit

Part Two Lunch Exchanges

3 protein
2 vegetable (10 grams)
1 fruit (15 grams) [this is optional]
total calories: 320

Sample Part 2 Lunch Menus

One 25-gram protein drink or drink mixed with 1 fruit or 6
    to 8 ounces fruit juice
Equals: 3 protein, 1 fruit

or

2 hard-boiled egg whites mixed with 2 ounces mock seafood,
    cut-up vegetables, chives, scallions, and fat-free mayon-
    naise. Spoon onto romaine lettuce leaves.
Equals: 3 protein, 2 vegetable

or

1 stuffed tomato*
Equals: 3 protein, 2 vegetable

or

$^1/_2$ cantaloupe filled with 3 ounces mock crabmeat salad mixed
    with 2 tablespoons parsley, 1 tablespoon dill, $^1/_2$ cup

*recipe on page 233

sweet red pepper, $^1/_2$ cucumber, 2 scallions, chopped, and 1
tablespoon fat-free French dressing
Equals: 3 protein, 2 vegetable, 1 fruit

or

chicken with pears*
Equals: 3 protein, 1 fruit

Snack

30 grams of a sweet or starchy carbohydrate totaling no more
than 140 calories.

Sample Afternoon or After-Dinner Snacks
(Choose *one* of the following selections)

10 rice minicakes, available in assorted flavors
1 cup fat-free caramel popcorn
2 large caramel rice cakes
$^2/_3$ cup Honey Graham cereal
$^2/_3$ cup chocolate Cheerios

or

100 calories of flat bread crackers, fat-free or low-fat,
cinnamon-sugar flavor. Check label for quantity.
Equals: 25 grams of carbohydrates

Dinner Exchanges

3 starch (45 grams)
2 vegetable (10 grams)
1 fat (5 grams)
total calories: 335

*recipe on page 232

Sample Dinner Menus

1½ cups Chinese-style noodles, 1 cup chopped
    mushrooms, onion, and bok choy, or chopped broccoli
    or asparagus
1 teaspoon sesame seed oil
Equals: 3 starch, 2 vegetable, 1 fat

or

1½ cups of potato baked with Shake 'n Bake roasted
    potato mix
1 baked apple
Equals: 2 starch, 1 fruit

or

zucchini frittata*
2 large pieces garlic bread (rub roasted garlic cloves on
    toasted French bread)
This meal has a small amount of protein
Equals: 1 protein, 2 starch, 2 vegetable

or

fresh asparagus and potato salad (see below)
Equals: 3 starch, 2 vegetable

RECIPES

Fresh Asparagus and Potato Salad

Best made in the early summer when fresh asparagus and tiny
new potatoes abound.

*recipe on page 233

Makes 2 generous servings

 3 cups tiny new potatoes, halved
 8 to 10 stalks fresh asparagus, cut into chunks
 2 medium tomatoes, diced
 $1/2$ cup sweet red salad onion, diced
 $3/4$ cup fresh string beans, cut into pieces
 $1/4$ cup fat-free garlic dressing
 2 teaspoons fresh oregano leaves, or $1/2$ teaspoon dried
 2 tablespoons fresh basil leaves, or 1 teaspoon dried
 freshly ground black pepper to taste

Put 2 quarts of water in a large saucepan; add the potatoes, and bring to the boil; cook 7 to 10 minutes. Add the asparagus to the water and cook an additional 3 to 4 minutes or just until potatoes are tender. Drain the vegetables thoroughly; empty into a large salad bowl and toss with the remaining ingredients. Marinate, covered, in the refrigerator for at least three hours or overnight.

Chicken with Pears

For a truly fabulous lunch, try this. It tastes equally good warm or cold.

Serves 2

 6 ounces skinless, boneless chicken breasts
 $1/4$ cup chopped onion
 $1/2$ teaspoon poultry seasoning
 $1/2$ cup low-sodium chicken broth
 $1/2$ cup evaporated skim milk or ready-made nondairy creamer
 16-ounce can pears packed in juice, not syrup
 nonstick cooking spray

Lightly spray a skillet with nonstick cooking spray. Cut the chicken into julienne strips and add to the pan. Stir-fry over medium heat until the chicken loses any pink color, 3 to 4 minutes. Add the onion, seasoning, and broth and continue cooking, uncovered, for 10 minutes. Add the milk or creamer and cook until broth is reduced by one third and slightly thickened. Add the pears and heat just until they are heated through. Note: If you prefer, puree the pears and use them to thicken the sauce.

Stuffed Tomato

If you're fortunate enough to have fresh herbs available, try the fresh thyme called for in this recipe. Otherwise try a squeeze of fresh lemon juice to enhance the flavor.

Serves 1

1 large beefsteak tomato
3¹/₂-ounce can tuna packed in water, drained
2 scallions, diced, including green tops
¹/₂ cup alfalfa sprouts
4 to 5 water chestnuts, chopped
2 tablespoons fat-free mayonnaise
salt and pepper to taste
fresh lemon thyme to taste (optional)

Cut the tomato in wedges, leaving the bottom intact, so that the tomato can be laid in a star shape on the plate.

Blend remaining ingredients and spoon over the tomato. Serve immediately.

Zucchini Frittata

A low-fat version of a classic.

Serves 1

2 egg whites
2 tablespoons chopped onion
$^1/_4$ cup chopped mixed green and red pepper
1 small zucchini, grated
1 tablespoon low-fat Parmesan cheese
nonstick cooking spray

Lightly spray a nonstick skillet with vegetable oil cooking spray. Beat the egg whites lightly; pour them into the pan, and cook over low heat until the eggs begin to set.

Mix the vegetables and cheese and sprinkle over the top; cover the pan and continue cooking until the frittata is puffed. Flip and brown one minute more. Serve immediately.

AVOIDING TROUBLE

1. Follow the plan precisely. Do not be casual about the timing of your meals or about eating the prescribed amounts of carbohydrate. Remember, if you have been following a diet that has suppressed the synthesis of serotonin, the transition from dieting to nondieting is as treacherous as tiptoeing through a minefield. As soon as you enter the battle zone of food choices, unrestricted meals, social dining, travel, and the necessity of preparing food rather than opening a ready-made diet meal or drink, you are in the presence of triggers that can easily and quickly destroy your eating control.

If you're concerned that once you have gone off the after-diet eating plan you won't be able to discipline yourself to eat at certain times of day, then after a week on this plan you should consider switching to the basic serotonin-seeker's diet. It will ensure sufficient carbohydrate intake from morning through night. If weight loss is no longer a goal, you can increase the calories on that plan by four hundred to six hundred, so that you will be eating between 1,800 and 2,000 calories a day. Consult the generic exchange table in Chapter Five for general information on the calorie content of each of the basic food categories, to help you figure out how many additional exchanges you can eat while staying within the new calorie total. But remember to keep your proportions constant. If you've decided to use up most of your additional calories at lunch, for example, and you eat six protein exchanges instead of the three on the diet plan, then you should also eat four starch exchanges instead of the recommended two (for a total of about 370 additional calories).

Note: Make sure you do not go on the serotonin-seeker's diet without first staying on the after-diet eating plan for a week. Only this plan will restore your abnormally low serotonin levels to the point where the carbohydrate portions (and proportions) allowed on the serotonin-seeker's diet will produce a feeling of satisfaction.

2. Give yourself time to adapt to the after-diet eating style, and bring the same level of commitment to this transition period that you brought to your diet. Remember your brain has ultimate control over what you do or don't eat—not diet books or counselors, spas or infomercials. Just because you temporarily turned over control to outside systems doesn't mean you can't repossess it. You can—and you will.

Many dieters claim that unless they go for weekly weigh-ins or participate in a program where their food logs are checked and they can talk about their problems to a sympathetic group, they cannot lose pounds or keep them off. It's true that support and monitoring help; when we're being watched we usually try harder—at least we generally do what we are told. However, the reason you are able to lose weight—supervised or not—is because you used your internal eating controls. If you had no internal controls, it wouldn't matter how many bionic women sang the praises of alfalfa sprouts, or how supportive your group was when you talked about your longings for chocolate milk shakes.

The reason you may now be apprehensive about regaining weight is, however, quite legitimate: Your diet has diluted your serotonin-fueled eating-control power. But the after-diet food plan will restore command to the rightful ruler—you. Once your serotonin system is fired up you will be able to depend on yourself without the aid of the additional support systems you used during your diet.

3. Remember to get plenty of exercise; it plays a critical role in the transition from weight loss to maintenance. If your calorie intake during your diet was very low—one thousand calories or less each day—you can be sure that your body drew upon the energy stores contained in your muscle tissue to compensate for calories not eaten. This, in combination with the fact that as you lose weight your muscle mass always decreases in proportion to the lesser demands being put on it, means that you lost muscle mass while you were dieting. That's a problem.

Muscle mass matters not just for strength but for calorie burning—a vital concern to anyone who wishes to lose weight or keep it off. The larger your muscles the more calories you will burn. As mentioned previously, this explains why men (who generally have larger muscles) lose weight faster than women.

I have seen this proven in a study at MIT. Men who ate substantially more calories than the women in the study still lost much more weight than the women—thirty to forty pounds compared with fifteen to twenty for the women. Measurements of body fat and muscle showed that the men had much less fat and more muscle both at the beginning of the study and at its end.

The only way to increase muscle mass, and therefore the rate at which your body uses up calories, is to exercise. If you are committed to keeping off the pounds you worked so hard to lose, exercise has to become part of your life. Without consistent physical activity the only way you can keep off the pounds is through constant, unwavering diet control, involving weighing, measuring, and counting every morsel of food you eat. Even if you slip up by eating just one hundred extra calories per day, you can find yourself gaining ten pounds a year.

Eating those additional one hundred calories a day is incredibly easy to do. A while ago a group of us at the Clinical Research Center at MIT were talking about a volunteer who was not losing weight as quickly as we thought she should. The dietitian mentioned that this woman was eating a large banana every day for one of her fruit exchanges. (One fruit exchange equals only *half* a banana.) "So what?" asked one of my colleagues. "I eat two bananas a day without even thinking about it." "Well," responded the dietitian, "then you are eating over two hundred calories." My colleague looked stricken. "No wonder I have been putting on weight," she said. "I've gained five pounds this year and I couldn't figure out why. The only thing I've changed in my eating is the number of bananas." The point here is not to vilify bananas but to show how very easy it is to accumulate extra calories through everyday choices.

Walking may be the most convenient type of exercise for you, and it's very effective. In a recent article published in *Obesity Research*, Drs. Ewbank, Darga, and Lucas found physical activity was extremely important in predicting whether ex-dieters would maintain their weight or regain it after a diet program was finished. The people in this study walked five days a week, with the most active covering a total of sixteen miles by week's end. All of them walked long enough to increase heart rates and body temperatures. Not surprisingly, the more they walked, the longer they kept off the weight.

If you can, find a friend or a small group with whom to walk; just make sure they are as committed as you are. If the weather in your area is not conducive to walking, consider investing in a treadmill—it's likely to cost less than your last diet program. Go to your local library, take out some books on tape, tune into your portable tape player, and walk. Listen to your favorite music and walk. If you are on a treadmill, stick a riveting movie in your VCR and walk. Start gradually, wear the proper footwear, and go at a slow pace until you build up strength.

Other exercises that are especially effective in the after-diet period are those that increase the large muscles of the upper and lower body. They include swimming, rowing machines, and the cross-country ski machines. Resistance training with machines and free weights will firm up arms, strengthen back and chest muscles, and tone hips and legs.

4. Don't give up your goal of maintenance if you cheat occasionally. Eating a couple of doughnuts or a high-fat meal is not an irrevocable mistake. Even if you gain two or three pounds, it doesn't mean you are going to regain thirty or forty. And it doesn't mean that you immediately have to return to that rigid diet program.

Do this instead. Follow the after-diet food plan for another week, or as long as it takes to suppress the temptation to dive mouth first into an all-out binge. Read Chapter Four to see whether some obvious or hidden stress is affecting your eating control.

If it is, then go to the appropriate food plan in this book. It will help to restore emotional stability along with eating control.

Exercise. As long as you are burning up some calories the damage will be minimized.

Stop feeling guilty. You're human—and you're in control.

CHAPTER TWELVE

Pharmacological Interventions: Redux

About ten years ago, as I was standing at the checkout counter of my local supermarket, my eyes were drawn toward the cover of a national tabloid newspaper (the kind with screaming headlines about alien babies). What caught my attention was the headline MIRACLE PILL CURES CARBOHYDRATE CRAVING.

With not a little trepidation I picked up a copy and was horrified to see my name—and that of MIT—featured in an article about a magic pill that would stop doughnut bingeing and melt pounds faster than ice cream on an August afternoon.

With my purchases—and the newspaper—in tow, I made a hasty retreat from the store, trying to figure out how an innocuous research paper I had recently published about a little-known drug had been transformed into a feature on a miracle substance that could cure overeating forever.

It turned out the MIT's customary press release on scientific findings had made its way into the hands of an intrepid reporter. However, rather than describing the sedate findings on a research drug that was able to reduce snacking on sweet and starchy foods by obese volunteers, the reporter had inflated our results into the best cure for obesity since famine.

Because that particular tabloid reaches millions of people, we were besieged by phone calls and letters from all over the country. Everyone wanted to know how they could get the drug. At that time my answer disappointed them: They couldn't, not even in France, the country where it was originally developed.

Today, things have changed. The drug is now obtainable in most countries throughout the world, including the United States and Canada, where hundreds of thousands of people are now using it to lose weight.

WHAT IS IT?

The scientific or generic name for the drug is dexfenfluramine. Its trade name in other countries varies, but in most places it is known as Isomeride and in the United States its name is Redux. And although it has not yet been shown to produce miracles, as the tabloid claimed it did, it does cause weight loss.

Dexfenfluramine aids the dieter in two ways, both of them stemming from their serotonin-affecting properties. The drug causes a feeling of fullness in the dieter almost immediately after he begins to eat a meal, and the drug also decreases the dieter's urge to snack on sweet and starchy carbohydrates. As we all know, feeling satisfied early on in a meal has a wonderful effect on controlling how much more we eat. In fact, the drug has been particularly useful for our subjects who had stopped smoking and who reached for second helpings and desserts instead of lighting up a cigarette at the end of a meal.

One research subject, a very overweight firefighter, could only stop eating when his stomach was so engorged with food that he experienced physical discomfort. This was a man who felt compelled to clean his plate every time he sat down to a meal. When he was home, he also ate everyone else's leftovers. Then he would help with the dishes by polishing off anything left in the pots.

Soon after receiving the drug (he didn't know what he was

being given), he told us that he was no longer able to finish the food on his own plate, much less anyone else's. He said he tried to eat more but couldn't. Even though he didn't feel stuffed he had to stop. Naturally he lost weight. And, just as important, the drug allowed him to understand—for the first time in his adult life—the difference between feeling satisfied and feeling stuffed. He learned that he didn't need to eat until he felt physically uncomfortable.

After the drug-treatment phase of the study was over we taught him how to capture that same feeling of satisfaction and fullness by eating carbohydrates rather than taking the drug. He was given an all-day food plan similar to the one described in the serotonin-seeker's diet (see Chapter Five).

DEXFENFLURAMINE AND EMOTIONAL DISTRESS

Dexfenfluramine is particularly effective at checking the impulse to devour excessive amounts of sweet or starchy snack foods when we feel emotionally distressed. As described in Chapter Two, we first learned this in the early 1980s in studies of obese volunteers who were using carbohydrates as edible tranquilizers. Those who were treated with dexfenfluramine halted their overeating and were able to regain control over their carbohydrate appetite.

We then extended our work to study people whose overeating was triggered by stress induced by physiological changes. We investigated using dexfenfluramine to control the overeating of sweet and starchy carbohydrates by women with premenstrual syndrome, patients suffering from Seasonal Affective Disorder, and ex-smokers. In all cases, the drive to ingest carbohydrates was propelled by the need to increase the serotonin stress-management system. And in all examples the drug decreased this overeating by enhancing the potency of the serotonin already in the brain.

HOW DOES DEXFENFLURAMINE WORK?

Like carbohydrates, dexfenfluramine reduces the appetite by working on the serotonin stress-management system, but it does this in a way quite distinct from carbohydrates. Serotonin, a neurotransmitter stored in certain brain cells until needed, becomes active when stimulated by other brain cells, leaves its storage place, and moves to a space between the cells. In this active state, serotonin is like a phone receiver with a working dial tone, ready to send messages. But after a short time, certain biochemical events occur that force serotonin back into the cells where it is stored. This reuptake of serotonin shuts off its activity as effectively as hanging up a phone breaks the connection.

Dexfenfluramine prolongs the transmission, or activity, of serotonin in two ways: by increasing the amount of serotonin that leaves the storage sites, which is known as enhancing the release of serotonin, and by keeping serotonin from returning back inside the cells too soon, which is called inhibiting the reuptake of serotonin. Both these processes result in making serotonin more effective. Now there is more of it available and more time for it to function.

How does this differ from what happens when you eat carbohydrates? Eating carbohydrates stimulates production of serotonin, which neither dexfenfluramine nor any of the other drugs like it can do. As soon as serotonin is made, it is immediately used for whatever function for which it is needed. On the other hand, carbohydrates cannot prolong the activity of serotonin. Only the drugs can do that. Also, if you are treated with a drug like dexfenfluramine, it keeps working for twelve or more hours. Taken twice a day, it will ensure twenty-four-hour coverage. Carbohydrates, however, exert their effect on serotonin for only three hours or so after consumption.

It's fascinating to see dexfenfluramine's appetite-inhibiting effect in action, both in and out of the laboratory. Recently I had an occasion to see it in a social context, when I had dinner with a woman friend from Switzerland—where the drug has been sold for several years. This woman enjoys a good meal and always asks to be taken to her favorite Boston restaurant when she's in town. She mentioned that she was taking dexfenfluramine because she had gained about forty-five pounds the previous spring and summer after a skiing accident had left her immobilized for months.

When the food was served she dug in like the rest of us, commenting on the interesting array of tastes and textures. However, about fifteen minutes later, I noticed that she had stopped eating with more than half her food still on the plate. When I asked whether something was wrong she looked sad and said, "I just can't eat as much as I used to. I think I am hungry when I sit down to eat, but after eating for a short time I lose my appetite. I really want to finish the meal because it tastes so good. But I can't. I feel too full."

I must add, however, that although dexfenfluramine does a good job of restraining overeating, if it suits your taste buds and desire to continue to eat, you will ignore how full you feel and continue to eat anyway. No drug can, by itself, change old eating habits if you do not want to change them. After years of studying people who have been treated with dexfenfluramine, I know there are times when people will continue to eat although they have no real urge to do so.

One striking example of this phenomenon was related by a client who had gone on a cruise. She told me that she forced herself to eat even when she wasn't hungry because she felt she had to take advantage of the many meals and snacks. "I paid for them in advance," she said, "and I wanted to get my money's worth. Sometimes I had to force the food down but I made myself because I knew it would be a waste of money if I didn't eat every meal that was served."

Celebratory occasions when you simply feel like letting go, nights out on the town when you have the opportunity to indulge in a fabulous meal, or long plane rides when you eat to relieve boredom—all these and many other causes can prompt you to eat much more than your body wants. Eating to fill time is a particularly hard habit to break, as I've seen with a number of volunteers in our study who did *not* lose weight on dexfenfluramine. Unwilling to give up their habit of nibbling when

faced with long boring evenings or weekends and often un-
aware of how much they were eating, they used the act of
putting food in their mouths to fill empty hours. So take note:
Although dexfenfluramine will make it easier to be content
with moderate portions of food—making it an ideal comple-
ment to a diet, especially to the food plans in this book—these
drugs are not miracle pills. They will work only if you are gen-
uinely willing to stop the types of overeating that are driven by
force of habit.

SHOULD YOU TAKE THE DRUG?

The FDA issued very clear guidelines for use of the drug. You
must be 30 percent or more above medically advisable weight, or
you must have diabetes, high blood pressure, elevated cholesterol
and triglyceride levels, or other medical problems that would be
improved by weight loss, even if you aren't considered obese. At
the present time, testing has shown Redux to be safe for use for
up to one year.

The decision whether to take the drug is up to you and
your physician. He or she will decide how long you can stay on
the drug. In some cases your doctor will weigh the risk of continued obesity against the risk of continuing on the drug for
longer than a year. In the past, weight-loss drugs—including
serotonin-based ones—were prescribed for a maximum of three
months, and for good reason. The drugs lost their effectiveness
after two or three weeks, and some drugs were potentially addictive, so short-term use was mandatory.

However, it is well established that dexfenfluramine is not
addictive. A panel meeting at the FDA in October 1995 recognized this and recommended that the drug be prescribed without the types of restriction placed on drugs that are thought to
have abuse potential.

Currently, the medical obesity treatment and research community feels that patients who need to go on a prolonged program for weight loss should receive drug treatment for as long as

it takes them to lose the necessary weight. Some of these experts also feel there may be a subgroup of obese people who need to be treated continuously so that they won't regain lost weight. Their argument is that some people can't maintain a medically desirable weight because they suffer from a disorder that makes regulating food intake practically impossible for them. These experts contend that, like people who must inject insulin for diabetes or swallow antihypertensive medication to combat high blood pressure, a certain class of chronically obese people must also be put on a lifelong course of drug treatment.

Many experts note it is not surprising that such people regain their weight once they stop taking their medication. They compare them to patients whose blood pressure soars if they go off their medicine. To them it's obvious: Medications work as long as they are taken. The FDA will allow dexfenfluramine to be prescribed for as long as two years and perhaps longer if future studies on lifetime effectiveness are carried out.

As more and more doctors prescribe Redux, they will expand on the information gained from research as to the best and most effective ways to use the drug. The problem with developing therapeutic recommendations from research studies and clinical trials is that research does not take into account the individual needs of the subject. For example, if an accountant is enrolled in a yearlong treatment study, yet really gains weight only in the high-pressure months of spring, he will nevertheless be treated with Redux for the entire year. Now physicians can work out the most optimal treatment plan for each patient and learn more about who is most likely to benefit from treatment.

To illustrate how a physician might use Redux differently for two different patients, let us look at the case of Sara and Simon. Sara, who was never overweight before her first pregnancy, found herself sixty-five pounds overweight after the birth of her first child. She shed about thirty of those additional pounds over the next eighteen months, then unexpectedly became pregnant again, gaining another seventy pounds. To help her lose the 105 extra pounds she is now carrying, Sara's doctor puts her on Redux for three months. Since Sara does not have an eating problem, and never had difficulty keeping her weight under control when she was not pregnant, her doctor used Redux simply to "jump-start" her dieting efforts. Sara went on to lose the rest of her weight on her own.

In contrast, Simon is treated with Redux for over a year. At 175 pounds overweight, Simon developed very high blood pressure and adult-onset diabetes. Even so, he refuses to seriously diet, scoffs at the idea of portion control and exercise, and pays no attention to what he eats, much preferring junk food to his wife's frugal, low-fat meals. On Redux, he was finally able to maintain a weight loss of about two pounds a month without any difficulty. His physician was not convinced, however, that Simon wouldn't revert to his old habits once the drug was stopped. So she decided that the health risk of keeping Simon on the drug (with careful monitoring) for a year after his weight loss was a much smaller one than the risk of having his blood pressure rise again or his diabetes get worse because he put the weight back on. Her hope was that Simon might become accustomed to his thinner body after the year and finally take some personal responsibility for keeping it that way.

WHAT ABOUT DOSAGE?

The dose, regardless of how much weight has to be lost, will probably be the same for everyone. This may seem an odd way to prescribe, but there is data to back it up. An extremely detailed and comprehensive study was carried out in this country in 1993 and 1994, verifying the effectiveness of the dose used in other countries where the drug is widely available. Subjects who received the smallest dose possible lost less weight but those given a higher than usual one did not have any more success than those on the already-established dose.

Like all drugs, Redux has side effects, most of which tend to disappear or diminish after a few weeks. The most common symptoms include diarrhea, dry mouth, and tiredness; the dry mouth may persist longer than the other two, and you will find yourself drinking more water than usual. Dizziness and abdominal pain have also been reported; the latter is considerably milder and much less common than what you might experience taking aspirin or the new over-the-counter drugs for pain and arthritis such as ibuprofen and naproxen. The Redux package insert carries a warning about a very rare but potentially fatal side effect called primary pulmonary hypertension (PPH). A slight increase in the incidence of this disease has been reported among people who have taken Redux and other weight-loss medications for long periods. The risk is statistically quite small, and it is important to note that obesity itself is a risk factor for PPH. But this risk underscores the importance of prescribing Redux as a drug to individuals with medically diagnosed obesity and not to those who simply want to lose a few pounds for cosmetic reasons.

THE BEST DIETS TO USE

Many doctors recommend protein diets to their patients who use Redux. While you will see some short-term results on these diets, in the long run protein diets will lower your stores of serotonin and make Redux less effective. Redux makes serotonin more active, but *it does not help the brain manufacture serotonin.* Only carbohydrates can do that. The best diets to use while you are taking Redux are those that increase brain serotonin. All diets in this book will work with Redux because they are all designed to boost serotonin levels in the brain; but if weight loss is your main goal, you will maximize the effectiveness of Redux if you start on the Serotonin-Seeker's Diet as soon as you start taking the drug. The action of the carbohydrates on this plan complements the action of Redux to ensure optimal serotonin activity.

During your first few weeks on the drug, you will notice that your appetite for carbohydrates has significantly diminished. This is because Redux specifically decreases appetite for sweet and starchy foods and increases hunger for protein foods. Potato chips lose their appeal and cottage cheese suddenly seems desirable. Don't be tempted by this sudden departure of your carbohydrate cravings to cut them out completely or even to restrict them significantly. Instead, use this period to try all those low or fat-free carbohydrates that you normally find unappealing. One patient felt so satisfied with rice cakes, popcorn, and other healthy carbs in the early stages of her Redux treatment that when she went off the drug, she found eating fatty carbohydrates like potato chips unpleasant.

Because Redux is so effective, many commercial weight-loss programs have started using it as part of their treatment regimens, without altering their traditional high-protein, low-carbohydrate diets. They do not offer food plans specifically designed to be used along with Redux. If you decide to join such programs because of the group or individual support they provide, follow their food plans only if they allow you to add in your essential carbohydrate snack and carbohydrate comfort dinner. Remove calories from other foods on the plan in order to do so if necessary, or re-arrange when you eat certain foods. For example, you might eat the packaged breakfast foods on the plan for your dinner since they are often higher in carbohydrate.

HOW MUCH WEIGHT CAN BE LOST?

The exact number of pounds lost depends, to some extent, on the amount that has to be shed. A very heavy person will lose much more weight during the beginning stages of any weight-loss program, with or without drugs, than someone who has fewer pounds to lose. However, according to the FDA, it is possible to predict whether or not a patient will lose weight at all on Redux by what happens during the first four weeks. In a twelve-month study about 80 percent of the patients lost four or more pounds in the first four weeks of treatment with Redux. These people went on to lose substantial amounts of weight during the rest of the treatment period—at least 10 percent of their total body weight was lost by the end of the twelve months. However, among those who lost less than half a pound a week during that first month, more than 90 percent of them lost nothing more during the rest of the program, even though they continued to receive the drug.

Redux, like all other weight-loss drugs, works best in combination with a diet, exercise, and, when needed, professional support or counseling. The best diet to follow is the serotonin-seeker's diet on page 64. You are holding it in your hand. The next thing to do is to figure out when and how you will exercise. Even though you will be spending less time eating, it's likely that you still will not have the time you need for exercise unless you change your schedule to fit it in. Why is it so important to do so? Because exercise keeps your metabolic rate from dropping as it normally does when you are losing weight.

As many of you know, when you go on a diet your body responds as if you were starving (which, in a way, you are). So your body goes into action to conserve every last calorie you are eating. The most effective way of doing this is to slow down the rate at which the body burns calories for energy—your metabolism. This is great if you are starving. For anyone trying to lose weight it's terrible.

A diet prescribing 1,000 or fewer calories per day has an even more extreme effect on metabolism, slowing it down much more than the higher-calorie plans found in this book. It may also cause your body to start burning some of the energy stored in its muscles, thereby decreasing muscle mass and further lowering metabolic rate. And the slower the metabolism, the slower your weight loss. Your muscle mass also decreases in response to losing weight, because your new, lighter body does not require as large a muscle mass to move it about as it did when you were heavier. This decrease in muscle mass is yet another reason your metabolism slows down. All these annoying obstacles to weight loss can be easily offset by exercise.

Start to exercise when you begin your diet and feel comfortable taking the drug. If side effects are a problem, then wait until they abate or disappear before engaging in any rigorous activity.

But as soon as you feel fitter and are losing weight, start a weight-training exercise program that will, at the very least, maintain your muscle mass. Increasing it, of course, would be even better. This is crucial if you have been a serial dieter in the past; each of your previous diets is likely to have left you with less muscle mass than before you began. The result can be particularly devastating to women.

Women begin their adult lives with less muscle than men, due to the lack of testosterone in their bodies. Women diet more frequently than men and are likely to decrease their muscle mass even further by their years of constant dieting. Thus, women's bodies can end up being composed mostly of bone, water, and fat, with very little muscle. While it's certainly not necessary to build the kind of muscles that would enable one to compete in a bodybuilding competition, women will find that working out with weights two or three times a week will rapidly increase the size of arm, back, and chest muscles, which in turn will cause the muscles to become speedier, more effective calorie burners.

A lot of people are intimidated by weight-training exercises, both the kind that employ free weights (barbells, for instance) and the kind that use machines to provide resistance. Either form of weight training requires some instruction. If you can, hire a well-qualified fitness instructor to work one-on-one with you to assess your level of strength and to design a program specifically for you. This can cost from thirty to sixty dollars for an hour-long session. Although this seems expensive, it is worth doing, especially if you have not exercised for many years. Certified instructors must go through a course and take a two-day national examination to obtain certification and must be recertified every three or four years. Before signing up with a fitness instructor, ask about his or her training, and ask to see a certificate or other credentials showing that the instructor has gone through a qualification program. A good trainer will show you how to breathe correctly (you would be amazed at how many of us breathe incorrectly while exercising), how to prevent injury, and how to hold your body to get the most benefit from the exercises you are doing. If you're working out on the machines at a health club or gym, you will also learn which machines work which muscles. Plan on a follow-up reevaluation four to six weeks later. You may have progressed so rapidly you can move on to a more intensive level of exercise. Don't, however, increase exercise intensity without supervision; otherwise, you risk injury.

Although you can get people to come to your house to give

you training in using free weights, the best way of getting yourself to exercise regularly—unless of course you are prepared to pay someone to come to your house weekly—is to join a sports facility. If the idea of signing up for a health club or gym appeals to you, be sure to check it out carefully before joining. Ask to observe or participate in a class so you get a feeling for the place. You want—and should have—an atmosphere that is sympathetic and understanding, and instructors who are competent and attentive. Visit a health club during its peak hour. If you feel that you won't be getting the care and attention you need, look elsewhere.

A less costly way of learning weight training is by renting several videos that demonstrate simple techniques. New videos appear often; the best way to choose one that is appropriate for your level of physical stamina and fitness is to sample several before buying. It is not necessary to invest in expensive equipment. For people who have never done weight training, especially women, all that is usually required to do it effectively is to use small weights, starting at two pounds and then, after these seem too light, increasing to five- or ten-pound weights.

SUPPORT

With or without a drug, dieting is hard, and many people find it easier to do with a partner or in a group. Sharing our "setbacks" with fellow dieters and exploring the reasons behind those setbacks often shores up our willpower and helps us stay on that diet another day, week, or month. Joining a commercial program is a choice that many of us make, except at this point, the Redux users are not segregated from the nonusers. So if you attend a meeting and share your experience on the drug, you may not find much interest among the group who are not taking it. Another option is to contact your state nurse's or dietitian's association and ask for the names of counseling nurses or dietitians in your area. These extremely knowledgeable and well-trained individuals might be interested in running Redux support groups in your neighborhood and allowing you the opportunity to meet with a trained health professional.

OTHER OPTIONS FOR WEIGHT-LOSS TREATMENT

The drug Prozac has become a household word in the last few years. It is one of several antidepressant drugs that treat mood disorders by increasing the activity of serotonin. Prozac and its first cousins Zoloft and Paxil, and the newer ones like Luvox and Effexor, are known collectively as SSRI, or selective serotonin reuptake blockers. These drugs act in a somewhat similar fashion as dexfenfluramine by prolonging the time serotonin remains active outside the cells. They are called reuptake blockers because they temporarily block the return of serotonin to the cells where it is stored. However, unlike dexfenfluramine, these drugs can't increase the amount of serotonin the cells push out of the cells in the first place. The drugs act only on what is there.

Do these drugs control overeating or aid in weight loss? So far, the answer is no. Initially, Prozac was regarded as a new weight-loss drug because patients who normally gain weight when depressed lost weight while being treated with it. It looked as if Prozac would not only help depression but also might be effective as a general weight-loss drug. Many clinical trials were carried out over the last eight years to test Prozac on obese people. At MIT we used Prozac in two research studies: a weight-loss study and an investigation into prevention of weight gain among ex-smokers.

While Prozac worked quite well in promoting weight loss in our obese subjects, we found it was not nearly as effective in preventing weight gain in former smokers. In the weight-loss study, the subjects steadily took off pounds over a three-month period; but in the ex-smokers' program the subjects started to gain weight fairly rapidly after only one month of treatment. Moreover, longer-term studies of Prozac have shown the weight loss enjoyed by our obese subjects was not likely to be long-lived either.

Other groups have shown that when Prozac is used for a full year, it causes a U-shaped pattern of weight change: During the first six months on the drug, pounds are shed; during the second six months weight is regained. Prozac is no longer considered a weight-loss aid.

PROZAC AND PMS: A PRESCRIPTION FOR WEIGHT GAIN?

Prozac, along with some of the other antidepressants like Zoloft and Paxil, has been shown to successfully relieve the mood disturbances of PMS, and it is conceivable that women treated with these drugs may also find their eating easier to control. Unfortunately, there is no information available on this in any of the studies published to date. Also, it is not yet known what the effects are on eating and weight gain or loss when, as is now the case, women with severe PMS take Prozac continuously for months or even years. If the year-long studies done on obese patients are any indication, the long-term result may be weight gain. But we don't know if the effect will be the same or not.

CHAPTER THIRTEEN

When Binges Happen: Controlling the Damage

In a perfect world filled with calm workplaces, perfectly behaved children, and endlessly understanding spouses, none of us would ever feel stressed to the point of brownie inhalation.

Regrettably, daily life isn't like that. It can't be; there are too many things that can go wrong, things that can overwhelm even the most dedicated follower of the food plans in this book. There will be times when, despite your best attempts to control your eating, you won't be able to. An extremely stressful situation will have you in its grasp, your feelings will be pushed to the max, and your eyes will seek—and find—food.

A bakery will materialize in your field of vision. Or maybe your particular oasis will be a fast-food restaurant, a pizza parlor, or an ice cream store. Maybe you will seize upon the leftover coffee cake from this morning's meeting, an untouched slice of birthday cake from a colleague's party, or that open bag of sour-cream-and-onion potato chips on your son's desk. Whatever the source of temptation, the next thing you know, the food is in your mouth.

Minutes later, as you are licking the icing from your fingers or inhaling the last crumbs from the plate, you moan, "Oh, no!

I've blown the diet." Despite having read this book, learned what triggers you respond to, and identified and followed the appropriate serotonin-boosting plan, you've once again succumbed to out-of-control emotion-driven overeating. At such times, you will inevitably wonder, "What am I doing? What's wrong with me?" Lapses of eating control are as inevitable as death and taxes. Do not let a binge be an excuse for ending your diet. Bingeing doesn't equal failure, and it should never be the justification for going off your diet.

Slow down. Something has happened in your life to loosen your control over your eating. You may be acutely upset because of a serious misunderstanding with a loved one; perhaps you are being so relentlessly bombarded with problems that you barely have time to catch your breath. The result is that your self-control just gives out. Take heart—you have not failed and you are not alone. Once you accept the principle that occasional lapses are inevitable, you'll understand that they're not fatal. Life—and dieting—can go on quite successfully after the binge.

Here are two examples. Let's begin with Wilma, whose story is likely to strike a chord with many women. "I knew that he was wrecking my life but I never realized he was also the reason I was such a blimp," she told a group of coworkers who were sitting around, discussing old boyfriends. "Then summer came. He got a job in California and I was alone. I decided this was the time to finally drop those twenty pounds that were making my hips resemble bumper guards. So I joined a diet group. And I was really into it: I weighed and measured foods, eating only the ones on the exchange lists. And you should have seen me in the supermarket with my tape measure, making sure the bananas and apples weren't too big. But then he came back for a visit—two days I now refer to as the weekend from hell. I had conveniently forgotten how obnoxious he could be. We spent the entire time arguing, and all he did was browbeat me with his half-baked law school legalese. And, on top of everything, he had the nerve to ask me when I was planning on going on a diet! It's too bad he never knew how close I came to attempting homicide—he was so self-obsessed he probably would have wanted me to hire him for the defense. When he finally left on Sunday I just blew it. I had planned to go right to the health club to work off my anger, but it just kept growing and growing. Instead, I got into my car and drove to a nearby mall, practically sprinted into the first pizza place I saw, ordered a large pepperoni pie, and took it back to the car to eat it. But while I gnawed my way through the first few slices I had a revelation. What I really wanted to chew up and spit out was him. After about ten minutes of nonstop eating I said to myself, 'Why am I letting that jerk get to me? He's ruining my life and my diet.' So I took the rest of the pizza, dumped it in the trash, drove home, picked up my gym bag, and went off to exercise. And I made the vow never to see him again. And I haven't."

It's just possible that Wilma's pizza binge might have been prevented had she not been on a strict diet for several weeks before the weekend from hell. Like virtually all diets, except the ones in this book, hers was a real serotonin depleter that had left her helpless before the intense anger she had felt toward her boyfriend. Stress on top of one of those diets is a recipe for bingeing.

And let's hear from Julia. "That had to be the worst week of the year. On Monday, my sister called to inform me she had finally decided to get a divorce. When she went through the most recent list of my brother-in-law's exploits, I wanted to skewer him. On Tuesday, I learned that a big proposal I had been working on day and night probably wouldn't get funded, and I was being assigned to another project that would cause me to forfeit weekends for the foreseeable future. Late Wednesday afternoon, when the office was empty and I was about to leave, my husband phoned to tell me that rumors were rampant in his office—several people were going to be receiving pink slips that Friday, and it was a good bet that he was going to be laid off. Mind you—the week was still young. That's when I lost it. I became so upset I wanted to pound the walls, screaming. As I was about to leave— since I was the last one out of the office—I checked to make sure the heating element under the coffeepot was turned off. That's when I noticed a half-full pan of brownies that someone had left behind. I looked at the brownies; they were calling to me in the universal language of chocolate. Now I have to tell you that I really don't like chocolate all that much. But I was riveted. I seized the pan, raced back to my office, sat down, and began stuffing those brownies into my face. Before I knew it the pan was empty and I was disgustingly full.

"You know what was interesting? I didn't even care that I had just inhaled about a zillion calories. I just sat there thinking, 'I needed that.' It actually felt like the right thing to do. There was no guilt whatsoever. I washed out the pan, put it back by the coffeepot, and went home. Of course, by the time I got there I felt awful because I wasn't used to eating so much fat and sugar, much less chocolate, at one time. So I skipped dinner and didn't eat again until lunchtime the next day. The binge was so unlike me that after I calmed down I gave myself a chance to think about it (but not the events that precipitated it). The only explanation was that I was seized by an emotion I couldn't control. I've had similarly intense episodes, feelings in response to really tragic events, like the death of someone close to me. Obviously, the context of this feeling was different, but the sensation was similar. Then, I had broken down, sobbing, overwhelmed by a wave of sorrow that swept everything else in its path. And then it passed. I was emotionally exhausted but at the same time sort of relieved as well. That's how I felt after I binged: exhausted and relieved."

What had happened to these women? In both examples they plummeted into a binge-eating situation sparked by overwhelming stress and, in Wilma's case, by unnaturally low serotonin levels after several weeks on a high-protein low-carbohydrate diet. And both times the woman recognized who or what was pushing her out of control. Wilma was able to halt her binge by looking closely at what she was doing and why. She realized there was a more effective way of responding to her erstwhile boyfriend than eating her way through a large pepperoni pizza. And Julia correctly perceived her brownie attack was an almost inevitable consequence of an unusually stressful week.

Furthermore, neither woman viewed her misstep as an excuse for further bingeing or said to herself, "Well, I've already blown it, so I might as well continue to stuff myself." In fact, just the opposite occurred. Wilma, after throwing away her unfinished pizza, went off to the gym. After her brownie feast, Julia went home and skipped dinner. For both of them the binge was regarded as a one-time episode, not proof of the futility of dieting or the inevitability of regaining weight. In short, they clearly understood what had happened and saw it as an isolated event caused by unique circumstances.

There is something else common to Wilma and Julia that was crucial to their emotional well-being: *They refused to feel guilty.* Rather than being angry with herself, Wilma was delighted that her overeating finally gave her the resolve to dump her boyfriend. Julia recognized she was in the grip of an emotional force that gave her no alternative but to do what she did. Neither felt as if she had performed a criminal act. There was no reason to feel ashamed. So they did not add to the stress that caused the binge in the first place by feeling they needed to punish themselves for overeating.

CAN BINGES BE PREVENTED—OR STOPPED?

Could Wilma or Julia have been detoured away from the overwhelming urge to eat? Maybe—if they lived in a perfect world. In Wilma's case, if a close friend or family member had called her soon after her boyfriend had left, she could have been distracted and vented her anger verbally. One of Julia's coworkers might have walked in before she attacked the brownies, or her husband could have called back with the good news that the rumors about the layoffs had turned out not to be true. Or even if he hadn't had good news, they might have had a heart-to-heart chat in which she could talk through her anger and helplessness at the events of the week. But neither Wilma nor Julia had access to personal support when they most needed it. They did have access to food.

When intense, unresolved, and unrelenting stress shatters our self-control, we may binge. Although the food plans described in the book make this less likely to occur because they are designed to boost and maintain serotonin levels, extreme emotional strain can place such overwhelming demands on serotonin that even these plans can't do the job.

The emotional force that sweeps a Wilma or Julia into a binge is staggering. I can only compare it to a child's temper tantrum. When a youngster is in the midst of one there is nearly nothing to do except wait it out. Having lost control, the child will continue screaming and kicking and thrashing about until the whirlwind of emotion passes and leaves him exhausted and, finally, quiet.

The binger's frenzied devouring of food is akin to an eating tantrum. Just as the child seems to be driven by some emotional energy force, so too is the binger at the mercy of an overwhelming compulsion. The eating won't stop until the force finally plays itself out.

But just as it may be possible to minimize the frequency of tantrums by making sure the child gets enough rest, food, and attention, it is also possible to decrease one's susceptibility to bingeing by building up one's immunity to emotional provocation. All of us are prey to actions and events that tax our emotional control and well-being. And, like an immune system that may be bombarded by one cold virus after another, after a while our emotional immunity breaks down, we feel extremely upset, and we may lose our hold on our eating.

To push this analogy a little further, think about this: Just as you can decrease your susceptibility to every virus going around the office by making sure that you get enough rest, fresh air, and nutritious food, you can decrease your sensitivity to every "emotional virus" by ensuring that your serotonin levels are adequate.

ANTIBINGE THERAPY

All the food plans in *The Serotonin Solution* restore and maintain brain levels of serotonin. But the most effective of all the serotonin-enhancing food plans is the one in Chapter Eleven because it is designed to restore serotonin reserves that have been severely depleted by dieting. You can think of this food plan as sort of an antibiotic to be used in critical eating situations. Like an antibiotic, the plan should be used for ten days (or for two weekends and one week). By that time, unless your troubles are as bad as Job's, you will have built up your serotonin reserves and emotional immunity enough to make you invulnerable to bingeing. (Obviously, if life continues to propel you from one stress to another, you should continue on the post-diet eating plan until you feel able to manage your stress without bingeing.)

If or when you find yourself unable to avoid out-of-control eating, try to be kind to yourself. Things happen. If you must binge, try to choose foods that will do the least caloric damage. I know this is hard to do in the midst of a whirlwind of eating, but even small alterations in what you pick will help to minimize the calorie effect.

Buy baked or fat-reduced potato chips rather than the traditional higher-calorie fried ones. Eat fat-free breakfast cereals instead of higher-fat granola. Don't order extra cheese, sausage, or pepperoni on the pizza. Get a double dip cone of frozen yogurt, not high-fat ice cream. Choose low-fat brownies smothered in fat-free chocolate sauce instead of cheesecake. When you have had enough food—*stop*. As with a temper tantrum, the energy that drives your eating may disperse before the food is gone. At that point just walk away from the food. The binge is over.

Follow the post-diet food plan in Chapter Eleven for the next ten days and then return to whichever of the book's food plans you were following before the binge occurred.

THE BINGE THAT WON'T GO AWAY

There are some stressful situations that simply won't go away. If they are of the kind that causes enormous amounts of emotional pain, feelings of helplessness, worry, sadness, or frustration, these chronic, unrelieved episodes of stress can make control over eating practically impossible. You have no psychological energy to spare for dealing with the problem of bingeing, because it's all tied up in the stressful situation.

Intellectually you know how to prevent yourself from bingeing, but you simply do not have the energy to take even the first step of turning to the appropriate chapter in this book. You say to yourself, "Forget it. There is no way I can bear to read about exchange lists and measurements while I feel as though I'm under siege. I have too much to deal with to worry about my weight and eating. Let me just get through this. I'll think about my weight later."

I encountered a classic example of this behavior in a subject who was enrolled in one of our studies on serotonin-boosting diet drinks. This volunteer had been taught what to eat when stressed, and when she encountered the predictable daily irritants that were part of both her work and home environments she was able to follow the food plan successfully.

Halfway through the study, however, her daughter had emergency surgery. When our subject came to see us a week later she had gained four pounds.

"What happened?" we asked. "Didn't the drinks work to prevent you from bingeing?"

She looked at us incredulously. "You mean you actually expected me to mix and swallow the drink in the middle of that ordeal? You must be joking. I was too stressed to even *think* about the drink. Once I knew my daughter would be okay I sat in her room and ate all the junk food I could buy in the hospital gift shop."

THE BINGE BREAKERS

What do you do when you can't stop the binge? There are three substances (I'm reluctant to grant them the status of foods) guaranteed to stop bingeing almost instantaneously. They are: maple sugar candy, Marshmallow Fluff, and GU (pronounced goo).

Maple sugar candy is sold in gift shops, specialty food stores, and occasionally supermarkets. Available in one-ounce pieces containing about one hundred calories, they are often shaped like leaves or little fingers. Made of maple syrup from which the water is removed, the candy is so intensely sweet that most people find the idea of eating more than one piece just about impossible.

Marshmallow Fluff is nearly as sweet. Two tablespoons of Marshmallow Fluff eaten straight from the jar will make you lose all interest in eating any more of anything.

GU has the consistency of toothpaste and, like it, is squeezed out of its container. It comes in various flavors, including chocolate, and consists mainly of glucose, flavoring, and thickening agents. To eat it, you rip open the single-serving pouch (one hundred calories each) and squeeze the GU into your mouth. As the glop coats your tongue and teeth you will reach for water, not food. (Look for GU in health food stores and athletic wear shops; it has not yet entered supermarkets.)

These snacks, composed mostly or completely of sugar, are the perfect serotonin boosters. They don't contain any fat or fiber, and the sugar enters your bloodstream very quickly once the food is eaten. They are something more as well: *binge breakers.* Their intense sweetness and gooey texture make them unpleasant to continue eating after the first few swallows.

I have had several clients who insisted that they could not stop eating once a binge began. None of them made it through more than two pieces of maple sugar candy before conceding defeat. If you know you will not be able to halt a binge even if your stomach is achingly full, I suggest that you keep an emergency supply of these binge breakers handy. The maple sugar candy and GU are the best for this since they come in single-serving portions and can be stored in a glove compartment, handbag, or suitcase. You may never need to eat these foods, so think of them as first aid, for emergency use only.

AVOIDING TROUBLE

1. Acknowledge the cause of your binge. Many bingers are unable or unwilling to admit to themselves that they are engaging in an eating tantrum. If they do, they resist pinpointing its cause. One woman I know had a stash of candy bars she ate when-

ever her anger at her children escalated to an unacceptable level. Because she starved herself after these events, she didn't have a weight problem, and she was so mortified about her binges that she never wanted to talk about them. Finally some other health problems forced her to confront her eating pattern.

In talking with me she described the overwhelming rage that drove her to retreat to her bedroom and eat. It was rage of such intensity and ferocity it appeared completely out of proportion to the events that seemed to precipitate it, as she herself readily agreed. Because I felt she had to understand the sources of her anger before she could change, I suggested she seek some psychological help for herself and her family.

After a number of meetings with a therapist, she realized it was herself—not her children—who was the real subject of her anger, and that her rage was related to her decision to become a full-time mother. She regretted her choice and felt consistently enraged. When her children were annoying or irritating, her anger grew to the point where she had to stuff her mouth with food to prevent herself from screaming—or even becoming violent. Thankfully, once she was able to look at her behavior objectively, she took steps. Now back at work part-time, she enjoys both her children and her career, and has her bingeing under control.

A binge should be followed by insight. The question the now-calm eater has to ask is, "Why did I eat that way? What is going on?" Wilma and Julia knew. But the stay-at-home mother did not understand what was triggering her distress and excessive eating until she received therapy. If you, too, feel unable to answer the question, then you might want to consider getting professional help.

2. Never deny that a binge occurred. And don't excuse it by telling yourself you lack willpower or are a hopeless overeater or are addicted to food. None of these things are true. Understanding your binge triggers gives you the power to overcome them the next time.

3. Make the binge self-contained. The binge can't be used as an excuse for further bouts of overeating or as a means of punishing yourself for losing control.

I remember a client I saw after she had completed a diet of several months' duration. She was suffering from a bad case of post-diet bingeing because she had been on a carbohydrate-free eating plan. Naturally she believed her frequent binge episodes were her own fault and she was furious with herself. Each time she lost control in a binge she would continue to ingest copious amounts of food for two or three days thereafter.

I was completely puzzled by this behavior until she finally confessed she wanted to punish herself. Making herself gain even more pounds by virtually force-feeding herself seemed like a fit punishment for the crime of bingeing.

A less extreme but much more common response to a binge is to use it as an excuse for eating foods denied on a diet. "I am obviously not going to lose weight after that food frenzy," you think, "so I might as well eat what I like for the rest of the day." And sometimes you take it one step further: "And since I am being so bad, there's certainly no point in exercising today."

Sorry, these just won't wash. Binges happen. But when they do there is only one valid response once they are over: Return to the appropriate food plan immediately. And start exercising as soon as your stomach feels empty enough to allow you easy movement.

4. Don't use alcohol to stop the binge. It may seem the sedative effect that alcohol has on some people would be an ideal binge stopper. It's not. Do not use alcohol to try to put the brake on unrestrained eating. You are putting yourself at risk of bingeing on *it*. Not only are you drinking lots of extra calories, but also you are losing even *more* control over your behavior. Think about it. Drinking is never a good prescription for achieving rational thought or behavior. So never try to use it as part of any strategy for achieving control over yourself.

5. Never starve yourself or purge yourself by either vomiting or using laxatives. Starvation and purging are both extremely dangerous. If you are engaging in these activities please seek professional help. There are many well-trained health care providers who specialize in eating disorders.

6. Get professional help for compulsive bingeing. The recom-

mendations in this chapter pertain only to *incidental* binge episodes, not those that occur several times a week with predictable frequency.

7. Do not eat and switch. If you find the taste of the binge-breaker foods so cloyingly sweet that you can manage only a few spoonfuls, do not switch to a salty or crunchy food in order to keep eating. I have known many people who will begin a binge with a sweet food and then go to a salty one, wash it down with several glasses of sugary soda, move on to a less sweet item like muffins, and finish up with a heavily sugared high-fat food like ice cream. Switching from one food to another prevents overused taste buds from shutting down, thereby making eating boring.

If you are unable to stop eating after one or two binge-breaker foods and find yourself eating until your stomach is totally stuffed, waiting until it empties somewhat, and then starting again, you may be a compulsive binger. If that is the case you should seek professional help.

ONE LAST WORD

Once your binge has ended, start using your food plan immediately. Don't feel guilty. You didn't do anything terrible, and tomorrow is another day.

Think of bingeing as like being caught in a huge thunderstorm: You're overwhelmed by the force that has caught you up in its grip, powerless to resist it. But inevitably the storm passes and the sun comes out again.

The binge, too, will pass—and you will be in control once again.

APPENDIX

Exchange Lists

Protein Exchange

1 exchange equals:

beef—lean cuts such as round, sirloin, flank steak, London broil, tenderloin, or stew meat	1 ounce
cheese, cottage, regular	$1/4$ cup
low-fat	$1/3$ cup
nonfat	$1/2$ cup
cheese, non- or fat-free	2 slices
cheeses, low-fat—skim milk mozzarella, ricotta, American, Colby or Monterey Jack	1 ounce
cocoa or hot chocolate mix ($1/2$ ounce packet with water)	6 ounces
eggs	1
egg substitutes	$1/2$ cup
egg whites	2
evaporated skim milk	$1/2$ cup

fat-free yogurt	1 cup
fish—fresh, frozen, or canned in water	1 ounce
Instant Breakfast (diet) made with 1 cup skim milk	1 cup
lamb—leg, steak, shoulder	1 ounce
liver—beef, veal, pork, or chicken	1 ounce
low-fat buttermilk	1 cup
low-lactose milk	1 cup
1% milk	1 cup
pork—lean cuts such as center cut chops, boiled ham, tenderloin, Canadian bacon	1 ounce
poultry—chicken, turkey, or capon without skin	1 ounce
sausage—lean turkey or chicken varieties such as breakfast links	1 ounce
shellfish—fresh, frozen, or canned lobster, crab or mock crabmeat, shrimp, mussels, clams	1 ounce
skim milk	1 cup
tofu	4 ounces
2% milk	$^3/_4$ cup
veal—all cuts except cubed or ground	1 ounce

vegetarian burgers (Available in supermarkets or health food stores. Be sure to check the labels and include the specified fat exchanges where appropriate.)

yogurt, nonfat	1 cup

Fruit Exchange

1 exchange equals:

$^1/_2$ cup of fresh fruit or juice *or* $^1/_4$ cup of dried fruit. Since fruits come in such a variety, the following list may be helpful in figuring out how much you should be eating.

FRESH OR CANNED

apple (2-inch diameter)	1
applesauce, unsweetened	$^1/_2$ cup
apricots, medium	4
canned	$^1/_2$ cup
banana (9 inches long)	$^1/_2$
blackberries	$^3/_4$ cup
blueberries	$^3/_4$ cup
cherries, large	1 to 2
canned	$^1/_2$ cup
figs (2-inch diameter)	2
grapefruit, medium	$^1/_2$
segments	$^3/_4$ cup
grapes, small	1 to 5
kiwi, large	1
mango, small	$^1/_2$
mandarin oranges	1
melon (all types)	$^1/_8$ melon or 1 cup cubed
nectarine ($2^1/_2$ inch diameter)	1
orange ($2^1/_2$ inch diameter)	1
papaya	1 cup
peach ($2^1/_2$ inch across)	1
canned	$^1/_2$ cup or 2 halves
pear, large	$^1/_2$
small	1
canned	$^1/_2$ cup or 2 halves
persimmon, medium	2
pineapple	$^3/_4$ cup
canned	$^1/_3$ cup
plum (2-inch diameter)	2
raspberries	1 cup
strawberries	$1^1/_4$ cup
tangerine ($2^1/_2$ inch diameter)	2

DRIED

apples	4 rings
apricots	7 halves

dates	2 medium
figs	$1^1/_2$
prunes	3 medium
raisins	2 tablespoons

JUICE
apple juice or cider	$^1/_2$ cup
cranberry juice cocktail	$^1/_3$ cup
sugar-free	$^3/_4$ cup
grapefruit juice	$^1/_2$ cup
orange juice	$^1/_2$ cup
prune juice	$^1/_3$ cup

Starch or Bread Exchange

1 exchange equals:

bagel, small	$^1/_2$
barley, cooked	$^1/_3$ cup
beans and peas, cooked—black-eyed peas, kidney beans, baked beans in tomato sauce, black beans, split peas, chickpeas, lentils, pinto beans, and cowpeas	$^1/_3$ cup
biscuit, small	1
bran flakes	$^1/_2$ cup
bran nugget cereals	$^1/_3$ cup
bread crumbs	3 tablespoons
bread, diet type	2 slices
bread sticks (8 inches long, $^1/_2$-inch diameter)	2
brown bread	1 slice
bulgur, cooked	$^1/_2$ cup
Cheerios	1 cup
Chex type cereals	$^3/_4$ cup
cooked cereals—oatmeal, Cream of Wheat	$^1/_2$ cup

corn	$^1/_2$ cup
corn bread (2-inch cube)	1
cornmeal, dry	$1^1/_2$ tablespoons
corn on the cob (6 to 8 inches long)	1
couscous, cooked	$^1/_2$ cup
croutons	$^1/_2$ cup
dinner roll	1
English muffin	$^1/_2$
French bread (3-inch slice)	1
Grape-Nuts	3 tablespoons
grits, cooked	$^1/_2$ cup
muffin, plain, small	1
pancakes (4-inch diameter)	2
pasta, cooked	$^1/_2$ cup
pita or pocket bread (4-inch diameter)	1
plantain, cooked	$^1/_2$ cup
potato	4 ounces
rice, cooked	$^1/_2$ cup
rye or pumpernickel, thin slice	1
shredded wheat	$^1/_2$ cup
squash—acorn, butternut, winter	1 cup
tortillas, corn or wheat flour (6-inch diameter)	1
waffle ($4^1/_2$-inches square)	1
wheat germ	3 tablespoons
whole wheat or whole grain bread (thin slice)	1
yam or sweet potato	$^1/_3$ cup

Snacks

1 starch exchange equals:

animal crackers	8
crackers—rice, nonfat wheat, nonfat	

vegetable flavored, nonfat	
graham, matzoh	3
fat-free potato chips	1 ounce
oyster crackers (small)	50
popcorn, air popped or fat-free	
microwaved	5 cups
pretzels	$^3/_4$ ounce
rice cakes	2
Ry-Krisp	4
rusks	2
tortilla chips (nonfat)	12 to 14
zwieback	3

Vegetable Exchange

1 exchange equals:

$^1/_2$ cup cooked vegetables, 1 cup raw vegetable, or $^1/_2$ cup vegetable juice of the following (unless otherwise specified)

artichoke, medium	$^1/_2$
arugula	
asparagus, steamed	7 spears
bamboo shoots	
beans—green, snap, string, yellow	
bean sprouts	
beets	
bell pepper	
broccoli	
brussels sprouts	
cabbage	
carrots	
cauliflower	
celery	
cucumber, medium	1

eggplant
endive
greens, all types—collard,
    dandelion, mustard, turnip
kale
kohlrabi
leeks
lettuce, all types—iceberg, romaine,
    Boston, leaf
mushrooms
okra
rutabaga
spinach
summer squashes—spaghetti,
    zucchini, pattypan, yellow
tomato
turnips
water chestnuts

Fat Exchange

1 fat exchange equals:

avocado	2 tablespoons, mashed
butter, bar	1 teaspoon
whipped	2 teaspoons
cheeses, high-fat	$^1/_2$ ounce
cream, light	2 tablespoons
cream cheese	1 tablespoon
lard	1 teaspoon
margarine, regular	1 teaspoon
diet	1 tablespoon
nuts	$^1/_2$ ounce
oil, all types	1 teaspoon
peanut butter	1 tablespoon
salad dressings	1 tablespoon
light mayonnaise-type	2 teaspoons

mayonnaise-type	2 teaspoons
reduced calorie	2 tablespoons
seeds—pumpkin, sesame, sunflower	$^3/_4$ ounce
shortening	1 teaspoon
sour cream	2 tablespoons
sour cream, light	3 tablespoons

Condiments and "Free" Foods Exchange

1 exchange equals:

barbecue sauce	1 tablespoon
beverage or drink mixes sweetened with sugar substitutes	no limit
butter flavorings—Butter Buds	3 teaspoons
chili sauce	1 tablespoon
cocktail sauce	1 tablespoon
coffee, black	no limit
diet soft drinks	
garlic	1 head
gelatins flavored with sugar substitutes	$^1/_2$ cup
herbs, fresh and dried—parsley, basil, oregano, thyme, rosemary	according to recipe or taste
imitation bacon bits	1 teaspoon
ketchup	1 tablespoon
Molly McButter	1 tablespoon
Mrs. Dash Seasonings	no limit
spice blends—curry powder, cajun, poultry seasoning, Italian	
mustard	1 tablespoon
nondairy creamers	1 tablespoon
nondairy whipped toppings	1 tablespoon
nonfat mayonnaise	1 tablespoon
nonfat salad dressings	3 tablespoons
nonstick vegetable spray	to coat pan
no-oil salad dressings	2 tablespoons

picante sauce	2 tablespoons
pickle relish	1 tablespoon
pickles	$^1/_2$ cup
pimiento	according to recipe or taste
reduced-calorie salad dressings	1 tablespoon
salsa	$^1/_4$ cup
sauerkraut	$^1/_2$ cup
shallots	according to recipe or taste
soy sauce	1 tablespoon
steak sauce	1 tablespoon
sugar substitutes—Equal, NutraSweet, Sweet'n Low	no limit
Tabasco sauce	1 tablespoon
taco sauce	1 tablespoon
teas	no limit
teriyaki sauce	1 tablespoon
tomato sauce	2 tablespoons
vinegars—herb, white, cider, balsamic	no limit

Bibliography

Akerstedt, T. "Sleepiness as a consequence of shift work." *Sleep* 11 (1988): 17–34.

Arnow, B.; Kenardy, J.; and Agras, W. "Binge eating among the obese: A descriptive study." *Journal of Behavioral Medicine* 15 (1992): 155–169.

Atkinson, R.; Blank, R.; Schumacher, D.; Levine, J.; and Rich, D. "Combination drug treatment of obesity in a practice setting." *Obesity Research* 2, (1993): Suppl. 2, 82S.

Benowitz, N. "Pharmacologic aspects of cigarette smoking and nicotine addiction." *The New England Journal of Medicine* 319 (1988): 1318–1330.

Blomstrand, E.; Celsing, F.; and Newsholme, E. "Changes in plasma concentration in aromatic and branched chain amino acids during sustained exercise in males and their possible role in fatigue." *Acta Physiological Scandanavia* 133 (1988): 115–121.

Blundell, J.; Burley, V.; and Cotton, J. "Dietary fat and the control of energy intake: Evaluating the effects of fat on meal size and post-meal satiety." *American Journal of Clinical Nutrition* 57 (1983): 7725–7785.

Blundell, J., and Hill, A. "Serotoninergic modulation of the pattern of eating and the profile and hunger-satiety in humans." *International Journal of Obesity* 11 (1987): 141–153.

Bowen, D.; Spring, B.; and Fox, E. "Tryptophan and high-carbohydrate diets as adjuncts to smoking cessation." *Journal of Behavioral Medicine* 14 (1991): 97–109.

Bray, G. "Evaluation of drugs for treating obesity." *Obesity Research* 3 (1995): Suppl. 4, 425S–434S.

———. "Pharmalogic treatment of obesity." *Obesity Research* 3 (1995): Suppl. 4, 413S–418S.

Bray, G., and Delany, J. "Opinions of obesity experts on the causes and treatment of obesity—A new survey." *Obesity Research* 4 (1995): Suppl. 4, 419S–423S.

Bray, G.; York, B.; and Delany, J. "A survey of the opinions of obesity experts on the causes and treatment of obesity." *American Journal of Clinical Nutrition* 55 (1992): 151–154S.

Brezezinski, A.; Wurtman, J.; Wurtman, R.; Gleason, R.; Nader, T.; and Laferrere, B. "D-fenfluramine suppresses the increased calorie and carbohydrate intakes and improves the mood of women with premenstrual syndrome." *Obstetrics and Gynecology* 76 (1990): 2206–2301.

Bruce, B., and Agras, W. "Binge eating in females: A population-based investigation." *International Journal of Eating Disorders* 12 (1991): 365–373.

Caballero, B. "Brain serotonin and carbohydrate craving in obesity." *International Journal of Obesity* 11 (1987): 179–183.

Cowen, P.; Anderson, I.; and Fairburn C. "Neurochemical effects of dieting: Relevance to changes in eating and affective disorders." H. Anderson and S. Kennedy, eds. *Biology of Feast and Famine* 10 (1993): 269–284.

Darga, L.; Carroll-Michals, L.; Botsford, S.; and Lucas, C. "Fluoxetine's effect on weight loss in obese subjects." *American Journal of Clinical Nutrition* 54 (1991): 321–325.

Delgado, P.; Chaney, D.; Price, L.; Landis, H.; and Heninger, G. "Neuroendocrine and behavioral effects of dietary tryptophan restriction in healthy subjects." *Life Sciences* 45 (1989): 2323–2332.

de Zwann, M.; Mitchell, J.; Raymond, N.; and Spitzer, R. "Binge eating disorder: Clinical features and treatment of a new diagnosis." *Harvard Review of Psychiatry* 1 (1994): 310–325.

Endicott, J. "The menstrual cycle and mood disorders." *Journal of Affective Disorders* 29 (1993): 193–200.

Fernstrom, J. "Effects of the diet on brain neurotransmitters." *Metabolism* 26 (1973): 207–211.

Fernstrom, J., and Wurtman, R. "Brain serotonin content: Physiological regulation by plasma neutral amino acids." *Science* 178 (1972): 414–416.

Finer, N.; Craddock, D.; Lavielle, R.; and Keen, H. "Dextrofenfluramine in the treatment of refractory obesity." *Current Therapy Research* 38 (1985): 847–854.

Flegal, K.; Troiano, R.; Pamuk, E.; Kuczmarski, R.; and Campbell, S. "The influence of smoking cessation on the prevalence of overweight in the United States." *The New England Journal of Medicine* 333 (1995): 1165–1170.

Folkard, S.; Condon, R.; and Herbert, M. "Night Shift Paralysis." *Experientia* 40 (1984): 510–512.

Foret, J., and Lantin, E. "The sleep of train drivers: An example of the effects of an irregular work schedule on sleep." W.P. Colquhoun, ed. *Aspects of Human Efficiency.* London: Academic Press (1972), 273–282.

Fuller, R.; Snoddy, H.; and Robertson, D. "Mechanisms of effects of d-fenfluramine on brain serotonin metabolism in rats: Uptake inhibition versus release." *Pharmacological Biochemistry Behavior* 30 (1988): 715–721.

Garattini, S. "Biological actions of drugs affecting serotonin and eating." *Obesity Research* 3 (1985): Suppl. 4, 463S–470S.

Geliebter, A., and Aversa, A. "Eating in response to emotional states and situations in overweight, normal weight, and underweight individuals." *International Journal of Obesity* 15 (1991): Suppl., 39.

Giraud, D.; Martin, D.; and Driskell, J. "Plasma and dietary vitamin V and E levels of tobacco chewers, smokers and nonusers." *Journal of the American Dietetic Association* 95 (1995): 798–803.

Gold, P.; Vogt, J.; and Hall, J. "Glucose effects on memory: Behavioral and pharmacologic characteristics." *Behavioral Neural Biology* 452 (1986): 145–155.

Goldstein, D.; Rampey, A.; Enas, G.; Potvin, J.; Fludzinski, L.; and Levine, L. "Fluoxetine: A randomized clinical trial in the treatment of obesity." *International Journal of Obesity* 18 (1994): 129–135.

Goodwin, G.; Cowen, P.; Fairburn, C.; Parry-Billings, M.; Calder, P.; and Newsholme, E. "Plasma concentrations of tryptophan and dieting." *British Medical Journal* 300 (1990): 1499–1500.

Gormally, J.; Black, S.; Daston, S.; and Rardin, D. "The assessment of binge eating severity among obese persons." *Addictive Behavior* 7 (1982): 47–55.

Grunberg, N., and Straub, R. "The role of gender and taste class in the effects of stress on eating." *Health Psychology* 11 (1992): 97–100.

Grunberg, N.; Bowen, D.; Maycock, V.; and Nespor, S. "The importance of sweet taste and calorie content in the effects of nicotine on specific food consumption." *Psychopharmacology* 87 (1985): 198–203.

Grunberg, N.; Bowen, D.; and Morse, D. "Effects of nicotine on body weight and food consumption in rats." *Psychopharmacology* 83 (1984): 93–98.

Guy-Grand, B.; Apfelbaum, M.; Crepaldi, G.; Gries, A.; Lefebvre, P.; and Turner, P. "International trial of long-term dexfenfluramine in obesity." *Lancet* 2 (1989): 1142–1145.

Hall, J.; Gonder, H.; Frederick, L.; and Chewning, W. "Glucose enhancement of performance on memory tests in young and aged humans." *Neuropsychologia* 279 (1989): 1129–1138.

Hall, S.; Turnstall, C.; Vila, K.; and Duffy, J. "Weight gain prevention and smoking cessation: Cautionary findings." *American Journal of Public Health* 82 (1992): 799–803.

Hamburger, W. "Emotional aspects of obesity." *Medical Clinics of North America* 35 (1951): 483–499.

Heatherton, T., and Baumeister, R. "Binge eating as escape from self-awareness." *Psychological Bulletin* 110 (1991): 86–110.

Heitmann, B.; Lissner, L.; Sorenson, T.; and Bengtsson. "Dietary fat intake and weight gain in women genetically predisposed for obesity." *American Journal of Clinical Nutrition* 61 (1995): 1213–1217.

Heraief, E.; Burckhardt, P.; Mauron, C.; Wurtman, J.; and Wurtman, R. "The treatment of obesity by carbohydrate deprivation suppresses plasma tryptophan and its ratio to other large neutral amino acids." *Journal of Neural Transmission* 57 (1983): 1878–2195.

Jimerson, D.; Lesem, M.; Kaye, W.; Hegg, A.; and Brewerton, T. "Eating disorders and depression: Is there a serotonin connection?" *Biological Psychiatry* 28 (1990): 443–454.

Kayman, S. "Maintenance and relapse after weight loss in women: Behavioral aspects." *American Journal of Clinical Nutrition* 52 (1990): 800–807.

Kayman, S.; Bruvole, W.; and Stern, J. "Maintenance and relapse after weight loss in women: Behavioral aspects." *American Journal of Clinical Nutrition* 52 (1990): 800–807.

Klesges, R.; Meyers, A.; Klesges, L.; and LaVasque, M. "Smoking, body weight, and their effects on smoking behavior: A comprehensive review of the literature." *Psychology Bulletin* 7 (1989): 204–230.

Klesges, R., and Klesges, L. "The relationship between body mass and cigarette smoking using a biochemical index of smoking exposure." *International Journal of Obesity* 17 (1993): 585–591.

Kornhaber, A. "The stuffing syndrome." *Psychosomatics* 11 (1970): 580–584.

Kuehel, R., and Wadden, T. "Binge eating disorder weight cycling and psychopathology." *International Journal of Eating Disorders* 15 (1994): 321–329.

Lawton, C.; Burley, V.; Wales, J.; and Blundell, J. "Dietary fat and appetite control in obese subjects; Weak effects on satiation and satiety." *International Journal of Obesity* 17 (1993): 409–416.

Leibowitz, S., and Kim, T. "Impact of a galanin antagonist on exogenous galanin and natural patterns of fat ingestion." *Brain Research* 599 (1992): 148–152.

Leon, G.; Phelan, P.; Kelly, J.; and Patten, S. "The symptoms of bulimia and the menstrual cycle." *Psychosomatic Medicine* 48 (1986): 415–422.

Lewy, A.; Sack, R.; and Singer, C. "Treating phase-typed chronobiologic sleep and mood disorders using appropriately timed light." *Artificial Light Psychopharmacology Bulletin* 21 (1985): 368–372.

Lieberman, H.; Spring, B.; and Garfield, G. "The behavioral effects of food constituents: Strategies used in studies of amino acids, protein, carbohydrates and caffeine." *Nutrition Reviews* 44 (1986): 61–70.

Lieberman, H.; Wurtman, J.; and Chew, B. "Changes in mood after carbohydrate consumption among obese individuals." *American Journal of Clinical Nutrition* 45 (1986): 772–778.

Lissner, L.; Levitsky, D.; and Strupp, B. "Dietary fat and the regulation of energy intake in human subjects." *American Journal of Clinical Nutrition* 46 (1987): 886–892.

McTavish, D., and Heel, R. "Dexfenfluramine: A review of its pharmacological properties and therapeutic potential in obesity." *Drug Evaluation* 43 (1992): 713–733.

Marcus, M., and Wing, R. "Obese binge eaters: Affect, cognitions, and response to behavioral weight control." *Journal of Consultant Clinical Psychologists* 3 (1988): 233–439.

Menkes, D.; Coates, D.; and Fawcett, J. "Acute tryptophan depletion aggravates premenstrual syndrome." *Journal of Affective Disorders* 30 (1994): 2–15.

Monk, T. "Advantages and disadvantages of rapidly rotating shift schedules: A circadian viewpoint." *Human Factors* 28 (1986): 553–557.

Mortola, J.; Girton, L.; Beck, L.; and Yen, S. "Diagnosis of premenstrual syndrome by a simple prospective and reliable instrument: The calendar of premenstrual experiences." *Obstetrics and Gynecology* 76 (1990): 302–307.

The National Task Force on Prevention and Treatment of Obesity. "Towards Prevention of Obesity: Research Directions." *Obesity Research* 2 (1995): 571–584.

Noble, R. "A six-month study of the effects of dexfenfluramine on partially successful dieters." *Current Therapeutic Research* 47 (1990): 612–619.

Pomerleau, O.; Pomerleau, C.; Morrell, E.; and Lowenburch, J. "Effects of fluoxetine on weight gain and food intake in smokers who reduce nicotine intake." *Psychoneuroendocrinology* 16 (1991): 433–440.

Rapkin, A. "The role of serotonin in premenstrual syndrome." *Clinical Obstetrics and Gynecology* 35 (1992): 629–636.

Read, N. "Role of gastrointestinal factors in hunger and satiety in man." *Proceedings of the Nutrition Society* 51 (1992): 7–11.

Ribeiro, E.; Bettiker, R.; Bogdanow, M.; and Wurtman, R. "Effects of systemic nicotine on serotonin release in rat brain." *Brain Research* 621 (1993): 311–318.

Rosen, J.; Hunt, D.; Sims, E.; and Bogardus, C. "Comparison of carbo-hydrate-containing and carbohydrate-restricted hypocaloric diets in the treatment of obesity: Effects on appetite and mood." *American Journal of Clinical Nutrition 36* (1982): 463–469.

Ross, J.; Arendt, J.; Horne, J.; and Haston, W. "Night-shift work in Antarctica: Sleep characteristics and bright light treatment." *Physiology and Behavior* 57 (1995): 1169–1174.

Rossignol, A., and Bonnlander, H. "Prevalence and severity of the premenstrual syndrome: Effects of foods and beverages that are sweet or high in sugar content." *Journal of Reproductive Medicine* 36 (1991): 131–136.

Ryan, D.; Kaiser, P.; and Gray, G. "Sibutramine: A novel new agent for obesity treatment." *Obesity Research* 3 (1995): Suppl. 4, 553S–559S.

Sayegh, R.; Schiff, I.; Wurtman, J.; Spiers, P.; McDermott, J.; and Wurtman, R. "The effect of a carbohydrate-rich beverage on mood, appetite and cognitive function in women with premenstrual syndrome." *Obstetrics and Gynecology* 86 (1995): 520–528.

Schelling, T. "Addictive drugs: The cigarette experience." *Science* 255 (1992): 430–433.

Smith, S., and Sauder, C. "Food cravings, depression, and premenstrual problems." *Psychosomatic Medicine* 31 (1969): 282–287.

Spring, B.; Wurtman, J.; Wurtman, R.; ElKhoury, A.; Goldberg, H.; McDermott, J.; and Pingitore, R. "Efficiencies of dexfenfluramine and fluoxetine in preventing weight gain after smoking cessation." *American Journal of Clinical Nutrition* 62 (1995): 1181–1187.

Spring, B.; Wurtman, J.; Gleason, R.; and Wurtman, R. "Weight gain and withdrawal symptoms after smoking cessation: A preventive intervention using d-fenfluramine." *Health Psychology* 10 (1991): 216–223.

Steiner, M.; Steinberg, S.; Stewart, D.; Carter, D.; et al. "Fluoxetine in the treatment of premenstrual dysphoria." *The New England Journal of Medicine* 332 (1995): 1529–1534.

Stunkard, A. "Eating patterns and obesity." *Psychiatric Quarterly* 33 (1992): 284–292.

Stunkard, A. *A History of Binge Eating*, C. Fairburn and G. Wilson, eds. London: The Gilford Press (1993).

Torbjorn, A. "Sleepiness as a consequence of shift work," *Sleep* 11 (1988): 17–34.

Wadden, T.; Stunkard, A.; and Smoller, J. "Dieting and depression: A methodological study." *Journal of Consulting and Clinical Psychology* 54 (1986): 869–871.

Wallin, M., and Rissanen, A. "Food and mood: Relationship between food, serotonin and affective disorders." *Acta Psychiatry Scandanavica* 337 (1994): 36–40.

Walsh, A.; Oldman, A.; Franklin, M.; Fairburn, C.; and Cowen, P. "Dieting decreases plasma tryptophan and increases the prolactin response to d-fenfluramine in women but not men." *Journal of Affective Disorders* 33 (1995): 89–97.

Weintraub, M.; Hasday, J.; Mushlin, A.; and Lockwood, D. "A double-blind clinical trial in weight control: Use of fenfluramine and phentermine alone and in combination." *Archives Internal Medicine* 144 (1984): 1143–1148.

Weintraub, M.; Sundaresan, R.; and Schuster, B. "Long-term weight control study." I-VIII. *Clinical Pharmacology Therapy* 51 (1992): 581–646.

White, J., and Wolraich, M. "Effect of sugar on behavior and mental performance." *American Journal of Clinical Nutrition* 62 (1995): 242S.–249S.

Wurtman, J.; Brezezinski, A.; Wurtman, R.; and Laferrere, B. "Effect of nutrient intake on premenstrual depression." *American Journal of Obstetrics and Gynecology* 161 (1989): 1228–1234.

Young, S.; Smith, S.; and Pihl, R. "Tryptophan depletion causes a rapid lowering of mood in normal males." *Psychopharmacology* 87 (1985): 173–177.

Index

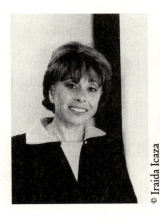
© Iraida Icaza

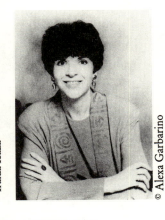
© Alexa Garbarino

ABOUT THE AUTHORS

JUDITH J. WURTMAN, Ph.D., is currently continuing her clinical research at the Massachusetts Institute of Technology. She has received pre- and post-doctoral fellowships from the National Institutes of Health. She is the bestselling author of *The Carbohydrate Craver's Diet*, and the coauthor of *The Carbohydrate Craver's Cookbook* and *Managing Your Mind and Mood Through Food*.

SUSAN SUFFES is a senior editor at a large publishing house.